D0861994

TIPS

that could
Save Your Life

Tendril Press

DENVER, COLORADO

Library of Congress Control Number 2010926723
ISBN: 978-0-9841543-0-2 Paper

10 9 8 7 6 5 4 3 2 First Publishing: 2011
Manufactured in the United States of America on acid free paper

Published by Tendril Press™
PO Box 441110
Aurora, CO 80044
303.696.9227

Author Photo by: Chris Roberts

Art Direction, Book and Cover Design
Copyright © 2010. by A J Images, Inc., All Rights Reserved
A. J. Business Design & Publishing Center, Inc.
A. J. Images, Inc. Communication Design
www.ajimagesinc.com
info@ajimagesinc.com — 303•696•9227

*The challenge to help the many
who are ill is to find faster,
easier, safer, more inexpensive,
and more effective ways to treat them.
Prevention is the first step,
and that is what this book is all about.*

Doris J. Rapp, M.D.

If you want to change the world,
be that change.

—Mahatma Gandhi

Contents

Appendix I: Harmful Chemicals and Where You May Find Them

Preface

This book was created because of my serious concern about the consequences of our ever increasing neglect of the health of our families, especially the next generation, and our planet. We simply cannot continue to allow excessive toxic pollution of our air, food, water, homes, schools, and workplaces. In one study, the newborns had an average of 287 toxic chemicals in their blood and urine. (Swann, U of Rochester) Their mothers have these same chemicals in their blood, urine, and even their breast milk. Some of these chemicals damage the brain and nervous system, the pancreas (causing diabetes), the thyroid (causing thyroid disease), the immune system (causing infection, allergy, and cancer), and the reproductive system (causing infertility and sex problems). Let's make some changes and give our newborns and everyone else a fighting chance.

We have increasing numbers of illnesses, some that never existed before, including ADHD, ADD, arthritis, autism, bipolar illness, cancer, diabetes, thyroid disease, obesity, infertility, Alzheimer's, neuromuscular diseases, etc. At times, all of these medical problems can be solely caused by exposures in our environment.

When will these epidemic-type illnesses stop? I do not believe this is possible until we all become much more informed about the causes and become proactive about the solutions. We know many causes, but we must take more interest in the politicians that are making the decisions that can negatively impact our environment and, thus, ourselves. The toxic chemicals are clearly detailed in my book, *Our Toxic World, A Wake Up Call*. Chemicals provide some clear answers as to why a number of these illnesses are so rampant. This book details how each of us can pinpoint many causes and hopefully diminish or possibly stop many of the harmful health effects.

This book was written to help you make your own little nests safer and more secure for yourself and your loved ones.

We must strive to find faster, easier, safer, more inexpensive, and more effective ways to treat illnesses. Too many parents cannot even afford the nutrients their family requires. Some can be helped quickly by doing a one week Multiple Allergy Elimination Diet and installing an air purifier, such as Austin Air. The booklet entitled *A Fast Easy Allergy Diet for Behavior and Activity Problems* outlines this allergy diet that costs nothing and easily detects many food allergies in 1-2 weeks. An air purifier can be tried for a few days to see if it appears to help dust, mold, pollen, and chemical sensitivities. If it stops symptoms, it is worth the cost. If it does not help, it can be returned for a small fee within a month. How many could be helped if these two options are tried first, before any potentially dangerous drugs are recommended for any family that has known allergies?

It is sometimes very easy to pinpoint and document cause and effect relationships by reading my book *Is This Your Child's World* (800-787-8780). The book also describes the pros and cons of using Provocation/ Neutralization allergy testing and treatment. (see www.drrappmd.com) or (www.greenhealthmedia.com). We can make better choices, but only if we are informed.

The answer to many medical problems is not another overpriced toxic drug, even if it is covered by medical insurance. The answer is to find and eliminate the cause. If you have a nail in your shoe, the treatment is not a bigger bandage, but to pull out the nail. This book will help you find the "nails" in your environment and explain why it is so essential for you to make a few significant changes in your lifestyle.

Please, read with resolve to make your personal nest more environmentally safe for the well-being of yourself and those you love.

Doris J Rapp, M.D.

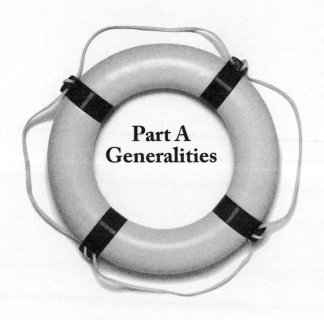

Part A
Generalities

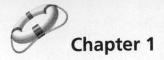
What You Drink and Eat

Tip 1: Water

Much of our home-use water is polluted and needs to be purified.

What Can You Do about It?

- A reverse-osmosis water purifier with charcoal is recommended.

- Install a water purifier or showerhead that removes chemicals in water used for showers and baths.

- Do not take long showers or baths in tap water unless you use a filter to help decrease toxins from the water or add detoxifying bath remedies such as Epsom salts, baking soda, or apple cider vinegar.

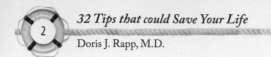

Read *Natural Detoxification*, Jacqueline Krohn, M.D., p261-p264.

○ Drink more pure water stored in glass or stainless steel (available at health food stores). Avoid drinking, storing, or freezing water or any other liquid in plastic, Styrofoam™, or aluminum. If you must use plastic, be sure that the recycling number on the bottom is #5.

○ Drink approximately half your weight in ounces of water per day in addition to two cups of pure water for each cup of coffee or other beverage. For example, if you weigh 120 pounds, you need sixty ounces, or seven to eight glasses of water per day.

○ Energized water with a correct pH balance is available. Read Robert Young's book, *The pH Miracle*.

○ Test your tap water for chemicals. For an inexpensive and accurate evaluation, visit *www.aquamd.com*.

Why is Purified Water So Important?

- Ground water makes up 50% of drinking water.[1]

  - Seventy-four toxic pesticides were found in the ground water in one study alone.[2]

  - Dursban is found in 25% of ground water. In some states, the levels can reach 65% in the spring when fertilizer or weed killers are used. This chemical can harm the kidneys, liver, and brain and cause birth defects.[3]

  - Atrazine contaminates 75% of stream water and about 40% of all groundwater in the Midwest.[4] It has been known to cause cancer in rats and sex deformities in frogs at 0.1 ppb (parts per billion). Atrazine in drinking water has been linked to leukemia, breast, and prostate cancer, and birth defects.[5] One million people drink water containing more than the acceptable EPA recommended safe levels of Atrazine, especially in the Midwest.

- Tap water can contain 141 or more unregulated chemicals.

- Millions of Americans drink water contaminated by toxic chemical fertilizers at levels above those which are known to be safe.[6]

  - Up to 60% of tap water can contain Triclosan, an antibacterial chemical found in soap. Toxic at 1 ppt (parts per trillion), according to the EPA's website, it is reported to cause increased perspiration, hormone problems, seizures, depression of the immune system, and cancer.[7]

  - A study published in September 2008 reports that 100% of urban streams sampled in California contained toxic levels of pyrethroids, the most common consumer-used pesticides[8] These chemicals can interfere with normal nervous system and brain function. High levels of exposure can cause dizziness, headache, nausea, muscle twitching, reduced energy, and

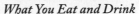

changes in awareness, convulsions, and loss of consciousness.

○ Tap water typically contains toxic fertilizers along with trace metals, drugs, contraceptives, antibiotics, and estrogenic mimicking chemicals, in addition to recycled sewage. Water treatment facilities can reduce the number of disease-causing germs in our drinking water. It is a challenge, however, to remove all the chemicals and prescription drugs found in human feces and urine. In other words, your drinking water can contain trace amounts of medications for high blood pressure, depression, cholesterol, hormone replacement, etc. Minute concentrations of some chemicals, even in ppq (parts per quadrillion), can cause drastic changes in how some people and animals feel and act.[9] What are we doing to ourselves?

○ Purified water has been reported to help prevent and treat illness. Drinking five glasses of purified water per day for six months is reported to decrease colon cancer by 45%, bladder cancer by 50%, and breast cancer by 80%.[10] Drinking ten glasses of purified water per day is said to decrease arthritis and joint pain after six months.[11]

Examples of People Who Suffered from Problems with Water:

<u>Mary</u>

Softened Water Causes Body Swelling and Hives

History:

- Mary first experienced hives at the age of ten years. By the time she was twelve, she suffered daily.

- She developed swollen joints and body swelling associated with extreme fatigue. Her knees became so swollen that she could not climb stairs. Her fingers swelled so much that her nails fell off.

⬭ Mary tried various medications, but found no relief.

Treatment: Dr. Rapp determined that Mary's symptoms began a month after her family installed a water-softening unit.

⬭ After discontinuing use of the water softener, Mary's symptoms quickly subsided.

⬭ When she accidentally drank some soft-ened water, she developed joint swelling that persisted for fifteen days.

⬭ Regular tap water did not cause this problem. She remained well as long as she avoided water that had been softened.

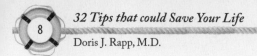
Tip #2: Other Beverages

Many common beverages create health hazards because they contain harmful chemicals and preservatives and because they are often stored or served in aluminum, plastic, or Styrofoam™.

What Can You Do about It?

- Avoid any beverage not stored in glass or stainless steel.

  - Drink large amounts of pure, clean water, organic juices, and organic herbal teas. Decrease or stop drinking any coffee (both caffeinated and decaf) and non-organic teas.

  - Do not drink "diet" beverages. See Tip 15: Artificial Sweeteners.

  - Avoid soda pops that list sodium benzoate or potassium benzoate on the label, especially if the drink contains citrus.

○ Do not drink beverages with the word "bromate" or "brominated oil" on the label.

Why Is It So Important to Be Careful about What You Drink?

○ Drinking beverages stored in aluminum is thought to contribute to Alzheimer's Disease.[12]

○ Benzoates can combine with citric acid to form benzene, which can cause cancer, according to the Federal Department of Agriculture.[14] Long-term exposure to high levels of benzene in the air has been linked to leukemia in children.[13]

○ Benzene is reported to cause anemia and damage to the immune system.[14]

○ Benzene is said to decrease the size of a woman's ovaries and cause irregular menstrual periods.[15]

○ The EPA (Environmental Protection Agency) classifies bromates as probable human carcinogens.[16]

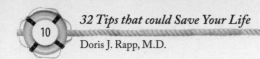

○ Ingesting bromate can cause vomiting, stomach pain, diarrhea, and hearing loss. Serious kidney damage also has been reported.[17]

Tip #3: Food

It is not how much you eat; it's your sensitivity to a food or beverage that determines if it is a problem for you. For some, a drop can cause illness, while others might require a cup or more before any symptoms occur.

Most foods are contaminated with chemicals unless they are organic. Approximately 25% of the foods in health food stores are not organic. About 25% of the foods sold in a regular grocery store are organic. In addition, many foods, particularly soy and corn, are now genetically engineered or irradiated, and this is a very serious concern.[18]

What Can You Do About It?

- Stop ingesting foods that obviously make you ill.
  - Eat only organic or pesticide-free foods or beverages as often as possible.
  - Eat mainly organic whole grains, brown rice, fresh fruits and vegetables.

- Eat foods that make your body more alkaline, such as *tomatoes, avocados, grapefruit, carrots, squash* (summer, butternut, yellow, etc.) *and green vegetables.* This will make your body less acidic and thus reduce symptoms of illness.

- If organic food does not fit your budget, consider the following suggestions:

  - Try growing your own.

  - Make friends with and offer to work for an organic farmer in exchange for fresh produce.

  - Join or work for an organic store co-op.

  - Create a community garden at church or in your neighborhood. Split the work and the crop.

- Chew your food longer and more completely. This helps to decrease allergies.

- Take digestive enzymes with each meal.

- Avoid genetically engineered or irradiated foods.

- Avoid consuming anything cooked or stored in aluminum.

○ Read nutritional labels and avoid ingredients that bother you. For example, foods that commonly cause allergies include milk and dairy, wheat, eggs, nuts, sugar, citrus, chocolate, corn, orange, artificial flavors, and dyes. Avoid these if they cause problems for you. Milk can be called whey or casein. Sugar can be called fructose or dextrose (corn sugar). Corn can be referred to as maize. Sometimes a label will say that it does not contain dairy, for example, but it contains such a small amount that it does not have to be listed. That small amount, however, can still cause allergies in some. See Appendix II for sources of some common allergenic foods.

○ Preservatives in food can be harmful. Watch out for propyl gallate. This additive may cause cancer and is often used with BHA or BHT, which have also been found to cause cancer. These are often found in cereal. The additive sodium nitrite (or nitrate) is found in bacon, ham,

14

hot dogs, and other processed meats and can lead to the formation of cancer-causing chemicals. For many years this chemical has been know to cause ADHD or hyperactivity.[19]

○ Eat meat with the lowest fat content. Chemicals are stored in the fat.

○ Notice how you feel, act, behave, breathe, and write or draw about fifteen to sixty minutes after eating. This is the best time to spot possible problem foods or beverages.

○ If regular food, such as a fruit, causes symptoms, but the same item purchased from an organic food store does not, it is probably the pesticides on or in the product that causes symptoms and not the food itself.

○ If you have symptoms of illness or some change in how you feel, act, or write before you eat, you may have low blood sugar or hypoglycemia. This often causes headache or irritability. If your symptoms

occur mainly within fifteen to sixty minutes after you eat, it is more apt to be food
sensitivity. Of course, you may suffer from
both problems.

- Read the excellent book entitled *Genetic
  Roulette* by Jeffrey Smith and Dr. Rapp's
  book, *Our Toxic World: A Wake Up Call*,
  Chapter Nine specifically, regarding
  genetically engineered foods.

Why is it So Important to Eat Healthy, Natural Food?

- Eating organic food decreases toxic
  substances in the blood by 50% in two
  short weeks.[20]

- Allergenic foods cause many unsuspected
  acute and chronic intestinal/bowel
  problems, including nausea, vomiting,
  bellyaches, belching, bloating, irritable
  bowel, Crohn's disease, diverticulitis, and
  ulcerative colitis.

- Some foods routinely cause delayed illness within six to forty-eight hours after
  eating. Symptoms include

- recurrent sinus, ear, or chest infections (often milk or dairy);

- bed wetting (often milk or fruit juice);

- hyperactivity (often dyes, sugar, milk, wheat, eggs, chocolate, corn);

- joint pain or arthritis (often citrus, yeast, tomato, mint, pork, beef, potato, bell peppers);

- colitis (often milk, wheat, chocolate);

- ulcers inside the mouth (especially in children, due to mint, tomato).

- Many are not aware that common foods can be the sole cause of the above types of reactions. For information about your symptoms, see Appendix II for a list of common problem foods and the symptoms they may cause.

- There are about 5000 preservatives/chemicals in our foods, and 2500 of them can cause cancer.[21]

- Toxic chemicals are reported to be in or on 25% of grain, 37% of fruits, and 34% of vegetables.[22]

- After artificial colors, flavorings, and the preservatives BHA and BHT were removed from school food in the 1980s, there was a 15.7% increase in academic performance.[23]

- Large amounts of Dioxin can be found in meat, dairy, chicken, and eggs.[24]

- Reports indicate that

  - One million Americans age five and under consume unsafe levels of a class of pesticides that can harm the developing brain and nervous system. Almost one in four peaches and one out of eight apples expose the eater to unsafe levels of pesticides.[25]

- Irradiation is often called "cold pasteurization" or "electronic pasteurization." According to the CDC, irradiation can change the quality of some foods. Meats with high fat content may develop an odor, egg whites can become milky or liquefy, raw oysters can die, and irradiated alfalfa does not seem to sprout as well. Nutritional changes due to irradiation include a "modest" decrease in some vitamins in the treated food, particularly B1 (thiamine).[26]

Examples of People Affected by Food Problems:

Kathie

History:

- ⚬ Kathie hiccupped and kicked in the uterus much more often than normal within a few hours after her pregnant mother ingested ice cream.

- ⚬ She was breast fed while her mother drank cow's milk.

- ⚬ As an infant, Kathie was overactive, extremely wiggly, and restless.

- ⚬ She slept poorly.

Treatment:

Kathie was seven months old when she came to see Dr. Rapp because of eczema. Her history suggested the infant was sensitive to something in ice cream. She was finally placed on a less allergenic milk formula, and she became calmer. With the newer form of allergy testing and treatment called Provocation/Neutralization, she improved. (Read *Is This Your Child's World?* by Doris J. Rapp, M.D., which discusses this testing in more detail). With treatment for foods and other substances, her eczema improved 75 to 95 percent and she became less anxious.

Triggers and Symptoms:

- Kathie's mother figured out that after she ate oats, carrots, or celery and then breast fed Kathie, the baby would develop eczema by the next day.

- When Kathie was tested, the milk allergy test triggered hyperactivity.

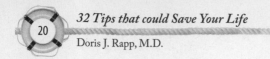

<u>Matthew</u>

History:

Matthew was an extremely hyperactive twelve-year-old boy whose behavior was impossible to control.

- As an infant and toddler, he only slept three hours a night and napped two hours a day.

- As he grew older, he developed leg aches, bellyaches, hay fever, and coughing.

- He was cranky, upset, and angry.

- He continually did somersaults and thumped and bumped around the rooms at school and at home. He never sat still.

- He had difficulty remembering.

Treatment:

He was placed on the Multiple Allergy Elimination Diet, and in four days, he was much better.* Within seven days, the improvement

*See DorisRappMD.com

was remarkable. He became less active and irritated, and he was friendly and happier. His aches and cough disappeared. After he was treated for his food allergies, his grades and behavior improved markedly.

Triggers and Symptoms:

- During the second week of the diet, it was determined that milk caused depression, irritability, and excess talking.

- Chocolate caused runny nose and bellyaches, corn caused excessive talking and insomnia, and red dyes caused stuffiness and "spaciness."

- Wheat caused listlessness and excitability. Once, he became so hyperactive that he started a fire in his basement and slid around in the water used to put it out. He was giddy the rest of the day!

- Sugar and eggs caused no symptoms.

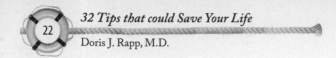

Scott

History:

- Scott, an eleven-year-old boy born into a family plagued by allergies, was very active as an infant. He broke his leg running into furniture as a toddler.

- He suffered abdominal pain and excessive belly gas.

- He experienced leg cramps at bedtime.

- Unpredictable and inappropriate behavior included irritability, grouchiness, clumsiness, restlessness, and hostility.

- He did not like to be cuddled or loved.

- School presented a myriad of problems for Scott. Besides his learning disabilities, he was easily distracted, had no friends, and fought with everyone. His behavior was even described as "insane."

Treatment:

- Scott was placed on the Multiple Allergy Elimination Diet.

- In one day, his cramps disappeared.

- In two days, his activity level was normal.

- Within one week, his mother said that her "bananas" kid was gone.

- He was able to play with other neighborhood children for the first time in his life.

- He became loving and kissed his parents.

- His belly gas and frequent crying were gone, and he was very cooperative.

- Successful treatment of Scott's food allergies revealed a pleasant personality that his mother had never seen before.

Notes

1. Kranz D, Kifferstein, B. "Water Pollution and Society." http://www.umich.edu/~gs265/society/waterpollution.htm (accessed June 28, 2010).

2. "Pesticide Contamination of Groundwater in the United States, Delaware Agricultural Experiment Station." *Journal of Environmental Science and Health*, 25, no. 1, (February 1990): 1-29.

3. *Toxic Chemical and Health*. A Summary of the Chemical Dursban. http://www.bhopal.net/oldsite/oldwebsite/hazdursban.html (accessed June 28, 2010).

4. Mae Wu, Mayra Quirindongo, Jennifer Sass, Andrew Wetzler. "Atrazine: Poisoning the Well : How the EPA is Ignoring Atrazine Contamination in the Central United States." NRDC, August 2009. http://www.nrdc.org/health/atrazine/default.asp (accessed April 27, 2010).

5. Kettles, M.K., S.R. Browning, T. S. Prince, S. W. Horstman. "Triazine exposure and breast cancer incidence: An ecologic study of Kentucky counties." *Environmental Health Perspective* Vol. 105, No. 11 (November 1997), http://ehp.niehs.nih.gov/members/1997/105-11/kettles-full.html (accessed April 27, 2010); Karla Gale. "Weed Killer Atrazine May Be Linked to Birth Defect." *Reuters* February 8, 2010 Health section. http://www.reuters.com/article/idUSTRE6174DW20100208 (accessed April 27, 2010).

6. Wang, Xinhao, Charlotte White-Hull, Scott Dyerm, Diana Mitsova-Boneva, and Mayura Ghode. "United States Drinking Water Quality Study Report." March 13, 2007. http://www.uc.edu/gissa/projects/drinkingwater/us_drinking_water_quality_project_report.pdf.

7. "Triclosan Fact Sheet." http://markey.house.gov/docs/triclosan_information_final.pdf (accessed June 28, 2010).

8. Holms, R. W., B. S. Anderson, B. M. Phillips, J. W. Hunt, D. B. Crane, A. Mekebri, and V. Conner. "Statewide Investigation of the Role of Pyrethroid Pesticides in Sediment Toxicity in California's Urban Waterways." *Environmental Science and Technology* 42 (2008): 7003-7009.

9. "Annual Water Quality Report." New York State. http://www.health.state.ny.us/environmental/water/drinking/annual_water_quality_report/docs/small_community_template.doc (accessed June 28, 2010).

10. "Water." http://www.zhealthinfo.com/water.htm (accessed June 28, 2010).

11. Frequency Rising. "Wellness for the Mind, Body and Soul." http://www.frequencyrising.com/water_dehydration.htm (accessed June 28, 2010).

12. Dr. Virginie Rondeau et al. "Relation between Aluminum Concentrations in Drinking Water and Alzheimer's Disease: An 8-year Follow-up Study." *American Journal of Epidemiology* 152, no. 1 (2000): 59-66, http://aje.oxfordjournals.org/cgi/content/full/152/1/59.

13. "Questions and Answers regarding safety of benzene in soft drinks." http://www.fda.gov/Food/FoodSafety/FoodContaminantsAdulteration/ChemicalContaminants/Benzene/ucm055174.htm (accessed April 28, 2010).

14. Shanghai, Shu XO et al, "A population-based case-control study of childhood leukemia." Shanghai Cancer Institute, Epidemiology Dept, People's Republic of China http://www.ncbi.nlm.nih.gov/pubmed/3164642 (accessed April 28, 2010).

15. "CAS# 71-43-2." Department of Health and Human Services Agency for Toxic Substances and Disease Registry.

16. "Bromate, CASRN 15541-45-4." IRIS, US EPA. http://www.epa.gov/iris/subst/1002.htm (accessed April 28, 2010).

17. "Bromate in Drinking Water - Information Fact Sheet." New York State Department of Health. http://www.health.state.

ny.us/environmental/water/drinking/bromate.htm (accessed April 29, 2010).

18. "Adoption of Genetically Engineered Crops in the U.S." ERS/USDA. http://www.ers.usda.gov/data/biotechcrops (accessed April 29, 2010).

19. "A Parent's Guide to Diet, ADHD & Behavior." The Center for Science in the Public Interest. http://www.cspinet.org/new/adhd_bklt.pdf (accessed June 27, 2010)

20. "Environmental Toxins." *Lancaster Health* http://www.lancasterhealth.com/index.php?id=environmental-toxins (accessed June 28, 2010).

21. "Pesticide Monitoring Program Report 2007." FDA.http://www.fda.gov/Food/FoodSafety/FoodContaminantsAdulteration/Pesticides/ResidueMonitoringReports/ucm169577.htm (accessed June 27, 2010).

22. id

23. Schoenthaler SJ, W. E. Doraz, J. A. Wakefield. "The Impact of a Low Food Additive and Sucrose Diet on Academic Performance in 803 New York City Public Schools." *International Journal of Biosocial and Medical Research* 8 no. 2 (1986): 185-195, http://www.feingold.org/Research/research_school.html.

24. Schecter, Arnold, P. Cramer, K. Boggess, J. Stanley, O. Päpke, J. Olson, A. Silver, and M. Schmitz. "Intake of Dioxins and Related Compounds From Food in the U.S. Population." *Journal of Toxicology and Environmental Health*, Part A, 63: (2001): 1–18.

25. "1 million American children age 5 and under consume unsafe levels of a class of pesticides that can harm the developing brain and nervous system." Environmental Working Group. http://www.ewg.org/node/20168.

26. Robert V. Tauxe. "Food Safety and Irradiation: Protecting the Public from Foodborne Infections." Centers for Disease Control and Prevention, Atlanta, Georgia, USA http://www.cdc.gov/ncidod/eid/vol7no3_supp/tauxe.htm.

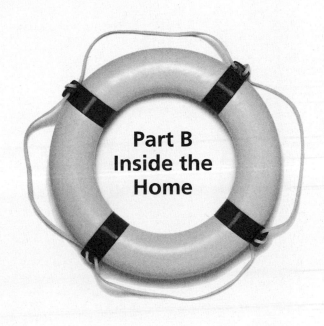

**Part B
Inside the
Home**

Chapter 2

General Tips for the Home

Tip 4: Household Cleaning

Many home cleaning products contain toxic
and harmful chemicals that can damage the
health of humans and animals.

What Can You Do about It?

- Avoid the following:
  - Ammonia
  - Dishwashing detergents
  - Drain cleaner
  - Toilet cleaner
  - Car wash solution
  - Grease removers

- Pine or cleaning products that contain toxic phenol

- Buy safer "green" cleaning agents:

  - Health food stores offer many varieties of "green" cleaning supplies.

  - For deodorizers as air fresheners, use citrus essential oils or ECCO mist.

  - For scouring powder, use Bon Ami, non-chlorinated products.

  - For disinfecting, use H_2O_2 (hydrogen peroxide). Visit *www.using-hydrogen-peroxide.com* for information.

- You can use baking soda and white vinegar for cleaning.

- A mixture of equal parts vinegar and warm water can be used as a glass cleaner. Vinegar is also excellent for cleaning chrome and removing lime buildup on bathroom fixtures.

- For candles, use only organic, natural wax and wicks.

- For drain cleaning:

- Pour one cup of baking soda down the drain, followed by one cup of heated vinegar. Five minutes later, pour in two quarts of hot water.
  Repeat several times if necessary.

- Laundry:

  - For bleaching laundry, use hydrogen peroxide.

  - Do not use regular fabric softeners. To soften fabrics, add one cup of plain baking soda to each load of wash.

Why Is It So Important to "Clean Green"?

- Fabric softeners can contain benzyl acetate, chloroform, and pentane. These can damage the lungs and brain and can cause cancer.[1]

- Solvents such as benzene, xylene, toluene, and styrene (Styrofoam™) can lower testosterone and sperm levels, as well as contribute to spontaneous abortion, birth defects, asthma, nose congestion, and can adversely affect the blood and heart. These chemicals are in many products but are erroneously not specified, but listed only as "inert" on the Material Safety Data Sheets. These solvents can be found in the blood and urine in many Americans.[2]

- Studies have indicated that dichloroben-zene (found in moth balls and deodor-ants) was found in the urine of 96% of children in Arkansas and in 98% of 1,000 tested adults across the United States.

- Ammonia can cause coughing, wheezing, nasal complaints, eye irritation, throat discomfort, and skin problems.

- Toilet bowl and drain cleaners contain corrosive alkalis and acids, which can damage skin and eyes.

- In one study on guinea pigs, mice, and chickens, all three species suffered from swelling and bleeding in the lungs after six weeks of ammonia exposure.[3]

- Pregnant rats exposed to phenols had excess saliva, rapid breathing, decrease in maternal weight gain, and underweight offspring. One in twenty-five mother rats died. The study authors attributed this death to the phenol treatment.[4]

- Exposure to formaldehyde causes eye, nose, and throat irritation, coughing, skin rashes, headaches, dizziness, nausea, vomiting, and nosebleeds.

- A formaldehyde study on rats showed decreased fluid intake and weight, as well as kidney and testes damage.[5]

Air Fresheners

Air fresheners can also contain toxic ingredients, including phthalates, acetone, limonene, acetaldehyde, formaldehyde, chloromethane, and 1, 4-dioxane.

What Can You Do about It?

- ♻ Use an oil warmer with a natural wax candle to warm essential oils and add natural, safe fragrance to your home.

- ♻ Stud an orange or grapefruit with whole cloves. You can make pretty designs and place them around the home, or combine a few clove-studded citrus fruits and some potpourri or wicker balls in a bowl for a beautiful and fragrant centerpiece. This is a great activity to do with children, as well.

- ♻ Simmer cloves, cinnamon sticks, or other whole spices in water.

- ♻ Place open containers of baking soda in the refrigerator, closets, laundry room, etc., to absorb odors.

Why Is It So Important to Use Natural Air Fresheners?

- ♻ Phthalates DEP and DBP, found in many air fresheners, have been linked to fertility and developmental problems in rats and have been banned from children's toys in twelve European countries. (CBC News)

○ Acetaldehyde is toxic when applied externally for prolonged periods. It is a probable carcinogen, it damages DNA, and causes abnormal muscle development.[6]

○ A study was done on top selling laundry and air freshening products at the University of Washington. All six products tested emitted at least one chemical regulated as toxic or hazardous under federal laws, but not one of those chemicals was listed on the product labels. (*ScienceDaily* July 24, 2008)

○ Chloromethane was used in the past as a refrigerant and was widely discontinued due to its toxicity to humans and animals.

○ In older refrigerators, exposure to chloromethane can result in dizziness, drowsiness, confusion, problems walking or speaking, and difficulty breathing, accompanied by gasping and choking. At higher concentrations, it can cause paralysis, seizures, and coma.[7]

- Formaldehyde causes cancer.[8]

- Dioxane is a form of ether and is classified as possibly carcinogenic to humans because it is a known carcinogen in animals.[9]

Tip 5: Indoor Air

It is now an accepted fact that indoor air can be up to *ten* times more polluted than outside air.[10]

What Can You Do about It?

- Check that your furnace/air conditioning filters fit correctly and change them monthly.

- Clean the ductwork in your home at regular intervals or, at a minimum, once every six months.

- Never allow any chemicals in your ventilation ductwork.

- Use a high quality air purifier.

  - Information on the pros and cons of air purifiers can be found by calling 1-800-787-8780.

- Use a high quality vacuum cleaner. To test your vacuum cleaner for dust leaks, turn it on in a dark room and shine a flashlight around it. Watch for dust particles.

○ Note if symptoms begin at times when the air conditioner comes on in the summer or when the furnace comes on in the winter.

○ Note if there is a fresh flare of symptoms whenever there is a change of season.

Why Is Clean Home Air So Important?

○ Improper air conditioning/heating filter care or chemicals in the ventilation system (HVAC) commonly cause chronic, perplexing illness.

○ Swamp coolers are not recommended because they are typically moldy.

○ Chemicals placed in ventilation ducts can be so toxic they never can be completely removed and can make a home or building permanently uninhabitable.

○ Some 30 million homes were treated with chlordane prior to 1988, when it was finally banned. There is a 75% chance you continue to breathe this chemical if your home was constructed prior to 1988. This chemical can persist for thirty-five years after application. The levels in a minute percentage of these homes, though very low, can continue to be dangerous and cause chronic illness.[11]

◎ Chlordane is reported to cause many common illnesses such as learning, emotional, mood problems, and even seizures.[12]

◎ A child sensitive to indoor and out-door air exposures.

An Example of Home Air Allergens

Darryl

History:

Darryl was "always" ill and wheezing. After checking his home, Dr. Rapp found that his bedroom was near an open door to a damp chemical-smelling basement. She urged the

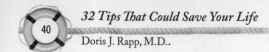

family to move, but their home had been in the family for two generations, and they could not afford another house. Allergy extract treatment helped, but Darryl continued to have sudden, severe episodes. He suffered whenever a lawn truck sprayed herbicides in the neighborhood or the wind blew from the Love Canal area of Niagara Falls, NY. He and his allergic neighbors all met in emergency rooms whenever nearby factories expelled their chemicals into the air.

Treatment:

An air purifier in Darryl's bedroom helped, but did not resolve the problem. His allergies improved when he moved out of his home. It is not unusual for children to believe they have outgrown their allergies when, in reality, they simply moved away from the source of their problem.

Tip 6: Mold

In addition to odor, there are numerous pervasive and often unrecognized symptoms related to mold exposures, spores, and the mycotoxins they produce.

What Can You Do about It?

- Eliminate any obvious water or plumbing leaks. Carefully review your homeowner's insurance plan to see if this type of problem is covered. The wording in policies can be very deceptive and misleading.

- If you have a sudden water leak, check the yellow pages under water damage and restoration. You may need to immediately vacuum up the water and place fans in the wet area to dry it out. Some firms are on call twenty-four hours a day. Fast action might make it possible to save wet carpets, providing they were water damaged for less than forty-eight hours. Of course, a plumber or roofer should be called to repair any leak.

- Use dehumidifiers, mold absorbers, and fans. These are helpful, but dehumidifiers must be cleaned very frequently. However, these measures are not adequate to resolve serious mold problems in buildings.

- Wash all moldy items with a good enzyme cleaner or EPA registered biocide. The Enzymagic 91 from *www.BestLivingSystems.com* is a 9:1 concentrate that sells for $43 a gallon. It produces 10 gallons of ready to use product, making it $1.45 a quart plus the spray bottle (another $2) for a total of $3.45 a quart. Regular household bleach does not kill mold. You need to use a more concentrated form called chlorinated bleach with a formulation that includes both sodium hypochlorite and sodium hydroxide. Also, some people are sensitive to the smell of bleach. Hydrogen peroxide can be used. It has no odor, but is not as effective.

- Do not use kerosene, formaldehyde, phenol, or pentachlorophenol to eliminate molds because they all can be too toxic.

○ Whatever you use must kill the mold and eliminate it completely. Simply stopping the mold from growing will not prevent sensitivities.

○ Some new products appear to effectively eliminate molds in the air and inside the walls, including the toxic mold called Stachybotrys atra. These organic, enzyme-based products can be forced through the walls into mold-contaminated areas, and should prevent the need for removal and replacement of walls, ceilings, or insulation. New products such as these might provide some major cost-effective applications for the remediation of heavily mold-contaminated homes, schools, and work places. Some moldy buildings are presently being condemned because they are not salvageable.
See *www.BestLivingSystems.com* or *www.Normi.org*.

○ With these products, significant mold spore reduction is apparently possible, and its effect can last for prolonged periods after only one application. Some mold-sensitive patients appear to improve within a few days.

○ Only preliminary research, however, is presently available, but these reports suggest this product can be most helpful. Environmental laboratories such as www.EnviroScreening.com continue to research new products for efficacy and their protective characteristics. Being in touch with trained mold professionals will help you get the latest and most accurate information regarding these technologies, sometimes even before they become commercially available.[13]

○ If you suspect a toxic black mold such as Stachybotrys atra, you might need advice from someone who has vast expertise in this field, as this mold can be very toxic. Contact experts in mold remediation

○ If you have mold sensitivities, the problem can be due to both a mold spore allergy and/or mold toxins (mycotoxins). These sensitivities usually can be detected by testing blood, nasal mucus, saliva, and lung secretions.

- The specific effects of mold spore exposure usually can be confirmed and treated rather easily by special allergy skin testing called Provocation/Neutralization. (Call AAEM 1-800-884-2236)

- Traditional allergy treatments can help most mold-related hay fevers or asthmas, whether seasonal or year-round.

- A new trichothecene mycotoxin urine or patch test has recently become available. This test is designed to help confirm the presence of a mold related illness and the need for mold remediation and treatment. You can order this test from *www.air-purifiers-superstore.com*

- Check your health food store for homeopathic remedies that claim to help alleviate mold allergy symptoms.

- *The Mold Source* is a website that can provide some important information. Visit *www.TheMoldSource.com*.

- NORMI, the National Organization of Remediators and Mold Inspectors, *www.NORMI.org*, has a place on their website where you can find qualified mold inspectors in your area, using your zip code. These professionals have taken solution-based training to help clients determine the source of mold issues and solutions.

- You can contact the American Industrial Hygiene Association to find the nearest hygienist who specializes in mold remediation. See *www.aiha.org*.

- Use a home mold test kit. There are some very inexpensive Mold Screening Kits and Pet Screening Kits available at *www.EnviroScreening.com*

Why Is It So Important to Do This?

▢ Certain air purifiers produce ozone. They appear to reduce both mold and germ contamination, and although many have used these machines and claimed to feel better, certain health concerns keep arising.[14]

▢ Because of ozone sensitivities at low levels and possible lung irritation from the smell of ozone, some recommend that ozone-generating machines be used only in areas where there are no humans, pets, or plants. After several hours of use, the windows and doors can be opened, and this should prevent or diminish mold or ozone-related health issues.

▢ Some believe there are no acceptable safe levels for ozone above normal outside air levels.

  ▢ Minuscule amounts that cannot be smelled unquestionably can cause some sensitive people to have definite respiratory distress. In addition, reports indicate that while ozone generators diminish certain airborne pollutants, they also may raise the levels of certain air contaminants such as formaldehyde.

- The American Lung Association recommends against negative ion generators because they are similar to ozone generators and can make some asthmatics worse. If you feel unwell from either ozone machines or ion generators, avoid them.

- Exposure to a damp, moldy environment appears to make chemical sensitivities, as well as the typical and less common forms of allergies, much worse. This "spiraling down" effect is all too common among those who first started out being allergic to only mold. Diagnosing and treating early is important.

Examples of Depression Due to Molds

Mike

History:

- In the late summer, when ragweed pollen and molds were a problem, this young man did not understand why he was so unhappy and depressed.

- He had no special health, school, financial, or relationship problems.

- His mother suspected he might have an allergy causing this problem.

Treatment:

When Mike came to see Dr. Rapp, he slumped and barely lifted his head. He avoided direct eye contact and was obviously very depressed.

One drop of mold allergy extract was placed on his arm. Within a few minutes, he began to sob. A weaker dilution of the same item

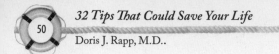
(Provocation/Neutralization allergy testing), brightened his mood within minutes. He remained that way and was radiant and joyful.

Amie:

At thirteen, Aime was a young lady who had the following reaction to one drop of a mold allergy extract. Before this test she was smiling and calm. Ten minutes after receiving a Provocation dose of mold extract, she rocked back and forth, developed abdominal pain, vision problems, and lethargy. She could write her name, but started at the end or middle, writing very slowly, as if unable to figure out which letter came next. After the Neutralization dose, she said, "Everything's ok now." She walked and wrote well with no problems.

Tip 7: Home Heating

Heating with natural gas, oil, kerosene, wood, or coal can all be harmful to your health.

What Can You Do about It?

- Use electric or solar heat, if possible, instead of gas, oil, or kerosene.

- Note if symptoms begin when the heat is first started at the change of season or when the blower on the furnace is in use.

- Check for gas leaks from hot water tanks, kitchen stoves, furnaces, or fireplaces, and always have them fixed immediately. Call the gas company. If they say they can't find it, call again, and continue to call until they have fixed the leak.

- Change/clean your furnace filter monthly.

Why Is It So Important to Use Electric or Solar Heat?

- ✿ Natural gas leaks can seriously damage human health and often cause chronic arthritis, learning problems, headaches, heart irregularities, and inappropriate activity and behavior.

- ✿ Certain types of coal contain arsenic, some in high levels. Chili peppers dried over coal containing high arsenic concentrations have resulted in thousands of cases of arsenic poisoning in the Guizhou Province of China.

- ✿ Kerosene is highly combustible and causes the buildup of carbon monoxide in closed spaces. In 1880, defective kerosene lamps caused 39% of NYC fires.

- ✿ Even as far back as the 13th century, British royalty banned the use of coal in London because of the harm to the quality of the air.

- ✿ In fireplaces, gas can continue to flow into the fireplace pilot light area after the switch has been turned to the "off" position, which is really just a disaster waiting to happen.

○ Wood and gas heaters emit nitrogen oxides and carbon monoxide. Nitrogen oxides cause breathing trouble and respiratory irritation. Carbon monoxide deprives the brain of oxygen, affecting brain function and consciousness. Carbon monoxide brain injury can be permanent. High exposure can cause death.

A Patient with Breathing Problems at Home Due to an Elusive Gas Leak: Sometimes You Must Check Things More Than Once

Shawn:

History:

Shawn exemplifies how mothers find answers. In my office this eight year-old boy always blew 300 on his PFM (Peak Flow Meter). A PFM is a simple instrument

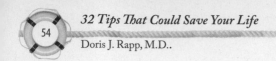

that is used to measure the ability to blow air from the lungs in asthmatic children. At home, however, he only blew 200. He wheezed every day when he was at home.

Treatment:

His mother said she smelled gas in the kitchen, but the gas company found nothing. The fourth time they checked her home again, they finally detected and fixed the leak. His wheezing at home stopped and Shawn could now blow 300 both at home and in my office.

Tip 8: Flooring

Linoleum, synthetic flooring, and some types of carpeting can be pesticide-laden and contain various chemicals that can be harmful to your health.

What Can You Do about It?

- Avoid smelly linoleum, soft vinyl, or synthetic flooring.
- Avoid moth- or stain-resistant carpets.
- In general, use hard tile, cotton throw rugs, or non-synthetic, natural carpets.
- See the video of the response of a mouse exposed to a synthetic school carpet on www.drrapp.com or www.greenhealth-media.com. The mouse becomes paralyzed in 3 hours and dies in four. Call (800)-787-8780.

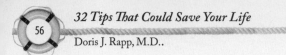

Why Is Quality, Chemical-free Flooring So Important?

- Synthetic carpets can have 4 phenylcyclohexene and styrene and butyl rubber in the backing.[15]

- The EPA put new synthetic carpets in their Washington, D.C., office in the 1980s. Over seventy employees had to be evacuated because of illness, and some continued to be ill and were unable to work because of the exposure.[16]

- Formaldehyde exposures in carpets are often unrecognized causes of asthma, hay fever, and recurrent infections such as flu, plus many other less-suspected behavior and activity symptoms.[17]

- Log cabins and wood decks or flooring tend to contain wood treated with toxic chemicals to control insects. These can include toxic preservatives such as creosote, pentachlorophenol and a chromated form of arsenic.[18]

An Example of a Patient with Sensitivity to Pesticide-treated Carpeting:

John

History:

John, age thirteen, had many allergies, as did others in his family.

- He returned to school one fall after extensive remodeling and the installation of new carpeting.

- He began to complain of his nose, tight chest, dizziness, headaches, nausea, and hives.

- His feet and joints ached, his ears felt full, and his voice was weak.

- He had a funny taste in his mouth. His fingers and lips tingled.

- His muscles ached, and he had dark circles and cramps.

- His arms and legs became progressively numb and tingly.

- By the end of the school day, he had double vision.

- His symptoms improved within one to four hours of leaving school or faded while he was on vacation. Shortly after he returned to school, his symptoms recurred.

- In addition, it was noted that within fifteen minutes of entering a newly painted or carpeted store, he experienced leg cramps and had to leave.

Treatment:

When he was tested with allergy extract made from air in his school, John quickly developed droopy eyes, extreme fatigue, and abdominal pain. The correct dilution of allergy extract quickly relieved these symptoms. His brain image changed, and this suggested that he possibly had been exposed to a toxin. This youngster continues to have to avoid chemicals in as many forms as possible and has detoxified his body in an effort to eliminate as many of the poisons as possible.

Tip 9: Furniture

The materials used in home furnishings can contain toxic chemicals such as pesticides and other irritants.

What Can You Do about It?

- Try not to buy plywood or synthetic filled or covered furniture.

- Use all natural wood, metal, or glass as much as possible.

- Try to find natural stuffing and covers. Organic cotton is preferred.

- Be cautious of wood furniture treated with preservatives such as creosote.

- Select environmentally-safe furniture.

- Avoid form-fitted, chemically-treated mattresses or pillows.

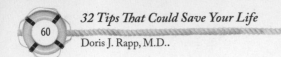

Why Is Avoiding Synthetic or Chemically-Treated Furniture So Important?

- Particleboard, fiberboard, and plywood often contain formaldehyde and other harmful chemicals.

- Many stores and manufacturers add pesticides or toxic chemicals to furniture to hinder the growth of mold and mildew.

- Creosote is a common wood preservative that can cause breathing problems, skin irritation, and cancer.

  - Both the International Agency for Research on Cancer and the EPA classify creosote as a probable human carcinogen.[19]

  - It is registered as a fungicide, insecticide, and repellent and is used to treat wood furniture. Skin contact can lead to intense burning and itching and may lead to chemical acne.

  - Skin and lung tumors occur in mice after skin contact with creosote mixtures.

○ Some furniture and textile fabrics are dyed with benzene or hydrazine. Benzene is a carcinogen and hydrazine is a probable carcinogen. Both can be extremely harmful to the body.[20]

○ Wood patio furniture may be heavily laden with pesticides. Metal or plastic is better.

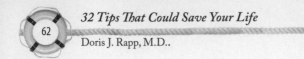
Tip 10: Pets

While you are keeping yourself healthy, don't forget to protect the health of your pets. Some pet foods can be hazardous to your animal, and flea collars and flea baths contain pesticides harmful to both pets and humans.

What Can You Do about It?

- Do not buy pet food that contains ethoxyquin. Use human-grade pet food.[21]

- Never feed dog food to a cat. Wet or soft dog food and dog treats can contain propylene glycol, which is harmful to cats.

  Try Flint River Ranch natural pet food, available at *www.FlintRiver.com*.

- Do not feed your dogs or cats grapes or raisins (possible kidney toxin), onions or onion powder, chocolate, citrus, alcohol, vitamins with iron, milk, dairy, mushrooms, raw salt, sugar, or raw eggs.[22]
  Give only large knuckle bones for chewing—others may splinter.

- Do not use flea collars or flea baths. Use a flea comb often, especially in the summer when fleas are at most prevalent.

- Instead of a flea collar, use a regular nylon collar and use essential oils such as citronella, rosemary, and rose geranium on it to repel fleas and ticks. **This is only for dogs, cats *cannot* tolerate the essential oils.** *Do Not Use Any Essential Oils on Cats!*

Why Is It So Important to Protect Your Pets?

- Ethoxyquin is added to pet food as a preservative, but it is also used as a pesticide.

  - The US FDA has found a verifiable connection between ethoxyquin and buildup of protophoryrin IX in the liver, which causes iron deficiency.[23]

  - It has been shown to cause mortality in fish.

  - Another problem is that eating food containing propylene glycol causes the formation of Heinz bodies in cats. These bodies damage red blood cells and cause anemia and are also associated with chronic liver disease. The use of propylene glycol has been banned in cat food, but is still used in wet dog foods and some dog treats.

- Eating onions also forms Heinz bodies in cats, as well as in dogs and some primates.[24]

- It has been reported that mothers who use an organophosphate flea shampoo (dichlorvos) on their pet during their pregnancy double the chance of brain tumors developing in their unborn babies by the age of five years.[25]

- Childhood brain cancer is five to six times more prevalent if flea sprays, shampoos, collars, or pest bombs/foggers are used in homes.[25]

- Bladder cancer is higher in dogs that have had certain flea and tick baths, and these baths may cause birth defects in their offspring.

Notes

1. "The Global Campaign for Recognition of Multiple Chemical Sensitivity. Could It Be Your Fabric Softener?" www.mcs-global.org.

2. Crinnion, Walter J. "Environmental Medicine, Part 2: Health Effects of and Protection from Ubiquitous Airborne Solvent Exposure." *Alternative Medicine Review* 5 (2000): 133-143.

3. Visek, Willard J. "Ammonia: Its Effect on Biological Systems, Metabolic Hormones, and Reproduction." *Journal of Dairy Science* 67 (1984): 481-498.

4. NAC/AEGL Committee. "Acute Exposure Guideline Levels (AEGLs). Phenol(CAS Reg. No. 108-95-2)." February 2006. http://www.umweltbundesamt.de/anlagen/AEGLWEB/Downloads/Phenol-full.PDF.

5. Til, H. P., R.A. Woutersen, V. J. Feron, V .H. M. Hollanders H. E. Falke and J. J. Clary. "Two-year drinking water study of formaldehyde in rats." *Food and Chemical Toxicology* 27 (1989): 77-87.

6. Environmental Protection Agency. "Acetaldehyde." www.epa.gove/ttn/atw/hlthef/acetalde.html (accessed May 6, 2010).

7. Agency for Toxic Substances and Disease Registry. "Chloromethane. CAS# 74-87-3." Agency for Toxic Substances and Disease ToxFAQs.

8. National Cancer Institute. "Fact Sheet: Formaldehydes and Cancer Risk." 2009. http://www.cancer.gov/images/documents/687f2693-82b5-4ec7-9c6f-e4e917d6ee53/Fs3_8.pdf (accessed May 6, 2010).

9. Environmental Protection Agency. "1,4Dioxane (1,4-Diethyleneoxide)." Revised 2000. http://www.epa.gov/ttn/atw/hlthef/dioxane.html (accessed May 6, 2010).

10. Mass, William. "Improving Your Home's Indoor Air Quality: From Basic to Bigger and Better Steps." 2009. http://greenhomeguide.com/know-how/article/improving-your-homes-indoor-air-quality-from-basic-to-bigger-and-better-steps (accessed May 6, 2010).

11. Offenberg, John H, Yelena Y Naumova, Barbara J Turpin, Steven J Eisenreich, Maria T Morandi, Thomas Stock, Steven D Colome, Arthur M Winer, Dalia M Spektor, Jim Zhang and Clifford P Weisel, "Chlordanes in the Indoor and Outdoor Air of Three U.S. Cities." *Environmental Science & Technology* 38 (2004): 2760-2768.

12. Sinclair, Wayne, Richard W Pressinger. "A Summary of Chlordane and Health Issues." www.main.nc.us/pace/11_archive_1/documents/summary.html.

13. Rea, William J. "Chemical Sensitivity." Vols. 1-4, 1992-1997. CRC Press, Boca Raton, FL.

14. National Toxicology Program. "Phenylcyclohexene [CASRN 4994-16-5]" Review of Toxicological Literature. 2002. http://ntp.niehs.nih.gov/ntp/htdocs/Chem_Background/ExSumPdf/Phenylcyclohexene.pdf.

15. Duehring, Cindy. "Carpet.Part One: EPA Stalls and Industry Hedges while Consumers Remain at Risk." http://www.holisticmed.com/carpet/tc1.txt (accessed May 6, 2010).

16. Home Air Purifier Expert.com. "You Are Probably Breathing Formaldehyde Right Now." www.home-air-purifier-expert.com (accessed May 6, 2010).

17. U.S. Department of Health and Human Services, Agency for Toxic Substances and Disease Registry. "Toxicological Profile for Wood Creosote, Coal Tar Creosote, Coal Tar, Coal Tar Pitch, and Coal Tar Pitch Volatiles." (2002) September http://www.atsdr.cdc.gov/toxprofiles/tp85-p.pdf.

18. Agency for Toxic Substances and Disease Registry. "Public Health Statement for Creosote." (2001) June. http://lldrm.org/assets/pubhealthstatementcreosote.pdf.

19a. Department of Health and Human Services, Centers for Disease Control and Prevention. "Chemical Emergencies Fact Sheet: Benzene." (2005) August http://lldrm.org/assets/pubhealthstatementcreosote.pdf.

19b. California Office of Environmental Health Hazard Assessment. "Chronic Toxicity Summary: Hydrazine." (2007) http://www.oehha.ca.gov/air/chronic_rels/pdf/302012.pdf.

20. Avianweb.com. "The Problem with Ethoxyquin." http://www.avianweb.com/ethoxyquin.htm (accessed May 6, 2010).

21. Drs. Foster & Smith.com. "Foods to Avoid Feeding Your Dog." http://www.peteducation.com/article.cfm?c=2+1659&aid=1030.

22. Drs. Foster & Smith.com. "Foods to Avoid Feeding Your Cat." http://www.peteducation.com/article.cfm?c=1&aid=1029.

23. Aldrich, Greg. "Ethoxyquin." (2007) http://www.petfoodindustry.com/ViewArticle.aspx?id=12892#Scene_1 (accessed May 6, 2010).

24. Beasley, V. "Absorption, Distribution, Metabolism, Elimination: Different Among Species." Ithica: International Veterinary Service Information, (1999) http://www.ivis.org/advances/Beasley/AppC/ivis.pdf.

25. Pagoda, James M. and Susan Preston-Martin. "Household Pesticides and the Risk of Pediatric Brain Tumors." *Environmental Health Perspectives* 105 (1997): 1214-1220, http://www.ncbi.nlm.nih.gov/pmc/articles/PMC1470343/pdf/envhper00324-0062.pdf.

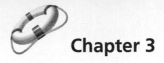

Chapter 3

The Kitchen

Microwaves, Teflon™ or aluminum cookware, and plastic are major concerns found in the kitchen that can seriously damage your health.

Tip 11: Microwave Ovens

These deplete the nutrients in foods and can cause serious health issues.

What Can You Do about It?

- Replace your microwave with an electric toaster oven for fast heating. They cost anywhere from $18.00 to $100. A toaster oven can save electricity and gas when used for small items that are normally cooked in a regular oven.

- If you must use a microwave, avoid using plastic wraps to cover food or beverages. Use a paper towel instead. Never heat any food or beverage in Styrofoam™ or plastic.

- Make popcorn on the stovetop using a ceramic or glass pot with oil, add the corn, cover, heat, and shake until the popping stops.

Why Is It So Important to Avoid Microwave Ovens?

- Microwaves ruin as much as 60 to 90% of the energy in foods, including vitamins B-12 and C.[1]

- One human study found that after eating microwaved food, hemoglobin levels decreased, causing anemia.[2]

- In 1991, an Oklahoma woman was killed when a nurse warmed blood for a transfusion in a microwave oven, which altered it. Blood is routinely warmed for transfusion, but not in a microwave. This shows us that microwaving is not the same as other methods of heating.[3]

- Microwave ovens can cause cataracts in humans. They can also cause digestive, liver, kidney, and brain damage.[4]

- At one time, Russia gave cataract prevention goggles with each microwave sold. After researching their biological effects in 1976, Russia banned microwave ovens; the ban was later rescinded.[5]

- Microwaving releases toxic chemicals from plastic or Styrofoam™.

- Microwaves have been reported to damage the digestive, excretory, brain, and nervous systems in both animals and humans.

- Many studies showed increased cancer cells in blood and organs.[6]

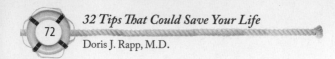

Tip 12: Non-stick Cookware

Studies indicate that Teflon™ (perfluorooctane, polytetrafluoroethylene, PFOA) and other non-stick cookware can damage your health.[7] (This does not include cookware with ceramic coating, which is non-stick, but does not contain the same chemical.)

What Can You Do about Teflon™ Exposure in The Kitchen?

- ○ Use glass, ceramic coated, or heavy stainless steel cookware. If cost is a concern, go to estate sales to find these.

- ○ Kitchen items often treated with Teflon™ or other non-stick coating containing the same chemical can include
  - Non-stick pots/pans
  - Woks
  - Utensils
  - Drip pans
  - Griddles
  - Non-stick baking sheets
  - Coffee makers
  - Electric skillets
  - Deep fryers and roasters
  - Waffle irons
  - Bread makers
  - Hot air popcorn poppers

- Never use these or any other nonstick cookware on high heat, especially near birds.

Why is Avoiding Nonstick Cookware So Important?

- Nonstick cookware surfacing (such as Teflon™) is made using perfluorooctanoic acid (PFOA), which is currently labeled as a likely human carcinogen by the U.S. Environmental Protection Agency. It never disappears and is very toxic to birds.[8]

- Chemicals released from hot nonstick cookware can contribute to indoor air and body pollution.[9]

- At least 90% of children and adults have PFOA in their blood. It is also found in most uterine fluid, breast milk, and the blood of most newborns.

- PFOA can cause flu-like symptoms in humans, including chills, headaches, and muscle aches.

- Some reports suggest that reproductive problems and delays in a child's growth and development can occur.[10]

- A small bird breathing nonstick coating heated only to 285 degrees can die within twenty-four hours.[11]

- It has been reported that living or working near or in a PFOA factory increases the chances of developing prostate and female reproductive cancers, as well as non-Hodgkin's lymphoma, leukemia, and multiple myeloma.[12]

- Reports indicate that PFOA causes rats to have smaller brains, damaged organs, and cancer.[13]

Tip 13: Aluminum

Aluminum can damage your health and has been linked to Alzheimer's disease.[14]

What Can You Do about Your Exposure To Aluminum?

- Stop using aluminum pots, pans, or rice cookers.

- Instead of aluminum foil, use an oven-safe glass or ceramic dish with a glass lid for oven cooking.

- Instead of covering foods with foil for heating, use paper.

- Do not use aluminum foil for food storage.

Why Is It So Important to Do This?

- Excess aluminum in the body cannot be processed, so it is deposited in various tissues, including the bones, brain, liver, heart, spleen, and muscles.

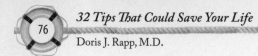

○ Aluminum can stay in the human brain for up to seven years before it is eliminated. This results in cumulative damage that could contribute to Alzheimer's Disease.[15]

Tip 14: Plastic

The chemicals present in plastic can cause serious damage to human and animal health, especially because of its sexual effects. (See Appendix I, Tables 4-7 for more information on plastics.)

What Can You Do about It?

- Try not to eat or drink anything stored in plastic. Use stainless steel or glass.

- Try to buy foods such as mayo, catsup, maple syrup, etc., in glass. If they are not available at your grocer, complain to management and insist that glass products be ordered.

- Store food items in paper (such as parchment or other paper made specifically for food), glass, stainless steel, or cheesecloth whenever possible.

- Avoid soft or smelly plastic.

- Do not heat, freeze, or store liquids or foods in plastic containers.

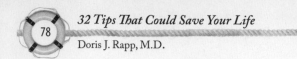

Why Is It So Important to Avoid Plastic in the Kitchen?

- Many plastic products contain BPA (Bisphenol-A) to strengthen the plastic. It is used in many baby bottles and food storage products, including the lining of most food cans.

- In April of 2008, Canada banned on the use of BPA in baby bottles. A U.S. senator then filed a bill called the BPA-Free Kids Act of 2008, which proposes banning the use of BPA in products that are intended for use by young children.

- Several states, including Wisconsin, Minnesota, and Connecticut have placed statewide bans on BPA.

- BPA has been linked to breast and prostate cancer, diabetes, hyperactivity, and other serious disorders in laboratory animals.[16]

- BPA causes early puberty in female rats and reduces fertility in rats.[17]

- Phthalates are plasticizers used to make plastic more flexible.

- Phthalates can be inhaled, ingested, and absorbed through the skin.

  - They cause precocious puberty in girls.

  - Phthalates can cause the male offspring of rats to become more feminine and to have abnormal reproductive organs, while the female offspring have more miscarriages.[18]

- Certain types of plasticizers found in the most frequently used types of plastic wrap (not polyethylene) can enter foods such as cheese and beef, either from direct contact or during microwave heating.[19]

- A plasticizer called nonyl phenol ethoxylate can cause inflamed vaginas in rabbits and appears to be able to alter their secondary sex characteristics and behavior.[20]

- Vinyl chloride (polyvinyl chloride) and ethylene chloride, found in synthetic plastics and cosmetic sprays, are similar in structure and effect. They can both cause liver, brain, intestinal, and kidney damage, as well as cancer in humans and rats.[21]

○ When plastics biodegrade, they release the greenhouse gas carbon dioxide. Burning non-biodegradable plastics also releases carbon dioxide. Disposing of non-biodegradable plastics in landfills causes the release of methane gas. When this gas finally begins to break down, it is even a worse greenhouse gas than carbon dioxide.

○ For more information on plastics, see Appendix I, Tables 4-7.

Tip 15: Artificial Sweeteners

Artificial sweeteners can cause serious damage to your health.

What Can You Do about It?

- Use stevia (liquid or powder) in place of saccharin, aspartame, or xylitol.

- It is much sweeter than sugar, contains no calories, and suppresses glucose response while increasing insulin levels. Some indigenous tribes in South America even use it to treat diabetes.[22]

- In Japan, where aspartame and saccharin are banned, stevia accounts for nearly 40% of the sweeteners on the market. It is marked as a dietary supplement in the U.S. due to federal regulations.

  - Do not drink "diet" or other beverages containing artificial sweeteners.

  - Carefully read labels on all "diet," "sugar-free," or "low fat" foods and

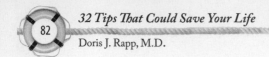

beverages that you purchase. These products often contain artificial sweeteners.

Why Is It So Important to Abstain from Artificial Sweeteners?

- ❍ Aspartame (brand name Nutra-Sweet®) damages the protective myelin coating of nerves, interfering with how the nervous system networks.[23]

- ❍ Recent studies in Europe show that aspartame use can result in an accumulation of formaldehyde (a known carcinogen) in the brain, which can damage your central nervous system and immune system and cause genetic trauma.[24]

- ❍ Aspartame has been linked with MS, lupus, and fibromyalgia and can cause headaches, migraines, panic attacks, dizziness, irritability, nausea, intestinal discomfort, skin rashes, and nervousness.[25]

- ❍ When aspartame reaches temperatures over 86°F, the wood alcohol in it converts to formaldehyde and then to formic acid.[26]

○ Aspartame is reported to cause weight gain, not loss.[27]

○ Splenda® is the brand name for sucralose. It is processed with chlorine, the idea being that the chlorine transforms the sugar molecule so it can't be digested; but there have been reports of up to 30% being absorbed by the body. Long-term use (several years) is reported to lead to immune system and brain disorders, but more research is needed to determine the extent of any possible damage.[28]

○ One report showed the combined use of Splenda® and aspartame depleted serotonin and caused insomnia for over a year until a doctor of homeopathy recognized the problem. Use of the sweeteners in this particular case also caused metabolism issues and weight gain.[29]

Notes

1. Mercola, Joseph, M.D. "The Hidden Hazards of Microwave Cooking." http://articles.mercola.com/sites/articles/archive/2010/05/18/microwave-hazards.aspx (accessed June 23, 2010).

2. id

3. Mercola, Joseph, M.D. "The Proven Dangers of Microwaves." http://www.mercola.com/article/microwave/hazards2.htm (accessed June 23, 2010).

4. "Jan Russell's Health Facts: Microwaving–Dangers to Your Food and You." http://www.jrussellshealth.org/microwaves.html (accessed June 23, 2010).

5. Gallawa, J. Carlton. "The Complete Microwave Oven Service Handbook" 2009. http://www.gallawa.com/microtech/Ch3.html (accessed June 23, 2010).

6. Wayne, Anthony and Lawrence. Newell. Health Freedom Resources. Public Announcement #2. June 2000. http://www.laleva.cc/environment/microwave.html (accessed June 23, 2010).

7. Costello, Tom. EPA: Compound in Teflon may cause cancer. 2009. http://www.msnbc.com/id/8408279 (accessed May 12, 2010).

8. "Is Teflon Risky?" *Time Magazine*, June 11, 2006. http://www.time.com/time/magazine/article/0,9171,1200779,00.html (accessed June 23, 2010).

9. Teflon and Non-Stick Cookware: Why We Should Not Cook With It. 2009. http://www.justlivegreener.com/living-green/greener-food-greener-cooking/84-teflon-and-non-stick-cookware-why-we-should-not-cook-with-it.html (accessed June 23, 2010).

10. Environmental Working Group. U.S. Toxics Registry Should Set Exposure Limit For Chemicals in "Teflon" Family. October 2009. http://www.ewg.org/ATSDR_Needs_To_Protect_People_From_Teflon (accessed June 23, 2010).

11. Doss, Joanne. "The Silent Killer." 2010. http://www. healthforwardonline.com/alt_health/Teflon/The_Silent_Killer_ by_Joanie_Doss.htm (accessed June 23, 2010).

12. Environmental Working Group. PFCs–Global Contaminants. http://www.ewg.org/node/21776 (accessed June 23, 2010).

13. Environmental Protection Agency (EPA). Preliminary risk assessment of the developmental toxicity associated with exposure to perfluorooctanoic acid and its salts. March 17, 2003. http://www.nicnas.gov.au/Publications/NICNAS_Alerts/PFOs_ Preliminary_Risk_Assessment_PDF.pdf

14. Alzheimer's Disease & Aluminum Connection. http:// www.moondragon.org/health/disorders/alzheimeralum.html (accessed June 23, 2010).

15. Bernardo, Jose F. *Aluminum Toxicity.* (October 2009) http:// emedicine.medscape.com/article/165315-overview (accessed July 2, 2010).

16 BPA and Human Diseases on the Rise. Environmental Working Group. http://www.ewg.org/node/20937 (accessed July 2, 2010).

17. Fernandez, M., "Neonatal Exposure to Bisphenol A Alters Reproductive Parameters and Gonadotropin Releasing Hormone Signaling in Female Rats." http://ehp03.niehs.nih.gov/article/info %3Adoi%2F10.1289%2Fehp.0800267 (accessed July 2, 2010).

18. Swan, S., "Chronic Di-n-butyl Phthalate Exposure in Rats Reduces Fertility and Alters Ovarian Function During Pregnancy in Female Long Evans Hooded Rats." (2000). http://toxsci.oxfordjournals.org/cgi/content/full/93/1/189 (accessed July 1, 2010).

19. "Plastic Wrap May Contaminate Food." *Midwest Today*, October 1999, http://www.midtod.com/plasticwrap.phtml (accessed July 3, 2010).

20. Nonyl Phenol and Related Chemicals "Inert" Ingredient Fact Sheet. Journal of Pesticide Reform, Spring 1996, Vol 16.1. http://www.pesticide.org/nonyl.pdf (accessed July 3, 2010).

21. Public Health Statement for Vinyl Chloride. Department of Health and Human Services, Agency for Toxic Substances and Disease Registry. http://www.atsdr.cdc.gov/toxprofiles/phs20. html (accessed July 3, 2010).

22. WebMD. "Stevia Uses." http://www.webmd.com/vitamins-supplements/ingredientmono-682-STEVIA.aspx?activeIngredie ntId=682&activeIngredientName=STEVIA&source=2 (accessed June 24, 2010).

23. Bowden, James and Arthur Evangelista. "Brain Cell Damage from Amino Acid Isolates." 2006. http://www.wnho.net/ aspartame_brain_damage.htm (accessed 2010).

24. Mercola, Joseph. "Study Links Aspartame to Lymphoma and Leukemia." July 2009. http://articles.mercola.com/sites/ articles/archive/2009/07/14/Study-Links-Aspartame-To-Leukemia-and-Lymphoma.aspx (accessed July 1, 2010).

25. Mercola, Joseph. "Aspartame: What You Don't Know Can Hurt You." http://www.mercola.com/article/aspartame/dangers. htm (accessed July 1, 2010).

26. id

27. Hull, Janet. "Ask Dr. Hull: Can Aspartame Cause Weight Gain?" Star. http://www.janethull.com/askdrhull/article. php?id=010 (accessed July 2, 2010)

28. Pick, Marcelle. "Sugar Substitutes and the Potential Danger of Splenda." http://www.womentowomen.com/healthyweight/ splenda.aspx.

29. Hull, Janet. "Ask Dr. Hull: Does Aspartame Cause Depression, Insomnia, Hyperactivity, and Mood Swings?" http:// www.janethull.com/askdrhull/article.php?id=020 (accessed July 2, 2010).

Chapter 4

The Bedroom

Tip 16: Mattresses and Bedding

Mattresses

Federal regulations presently allow boric acid, antimony, formaldehyde, or glass fibers to be used as flame-retardants. These are being used in and on any new mattresses and do not have to be listed on the label. In fact, the US government mandated that as of July 2, 2008, all new mattresses must be treated with flame retardant chemicals, but they did not mandate that these chemicals should be safe for humans. Flame-retardants are also used in many pillows, as well as crib mattresses.

What Can You Do about It?

- The box spring and mattress (or futon mattress) ideally should be organic cotton and have dust covers.

- Do not use urethane, polyester, synthetic, form-fitting, spongy, or smelly pesticide-laden mattresses or futons.
  To purchase a mattress that is guaranteed not to be treated with toxic flame retardant chemicals, obtain a note from your physician stating that you have a health problem that requires avoiding the use of toxic chemicals, and call 1-800-457-6442.

- If you can't afford costly organic cotton mattresses or pillows, you can make your own with layers of washed, organic flannel sheets. Sew the corner ends together and place it inside an organic cotton barrier cloth.

- You can also place several thick cotton blankets over a thick aluminum pad made from heavy aluminum foil on top of an old mattress. It can be noisy, but it is cost effective.

Why Are Natural, Chemical-free Mattresses So Important?

- Some urethane, polyester, synthetic, form-fitting, or pesticide-treated mattresses are so toxic that mice can develop breathing or skin problems, become paralyzed, and die within a few hours of exposure to the chemicals contained in them.[1]

- Flame retardant chemicals used on mattresses (and pillows) can contain boric acid (reproductive and developmental toxin, used as a pesticide), antimony (causes heart and lung damage, possible carcinogen), and decabromodiphenyl oxide (causes hair and memory loss, possible carcinogen).[2]

   - According to the EPA, the percentage of antimony present in most flame retardants is 27.5 times higher than the recommended safe percentage.[3]

○ One study indicated exposed workers
   in an antimony plant experienced
   a greater incidence of spontaneous
   abortions than a control group of
   non-exposed working women. A high
   rate of premature deliveries among
   workers in antimony smelting and
   processing plants was also observed.[4,5]

○ In 1994, Dr. Sprott of New Zealand said
   that fire retardants in mattresses combine with molds to make a gas that damages the brain and causes SIDS (sudden
   infant death syndrome). The central
   nervous system and lungs shut down,
   and the infant dies. Mattresses were then
   wrapped in polyethylene. In 100,000
   infants, no SIDS cases were noted. The
   control group (no polyethylene wrap
   on their mattresses) had 500 cases of
   SIDS.[6,7,8]

○ Vinyl on top of young children's mattresses will not prevent toxic exposures
   that can pass into the air.

Bedding:

Bedding such as pillows, blankets, sheets, and comforters often contain synthetic fabrics and/ or harmful, toxic chemicals, as well as many allergens such as dust and molds.

What Can You Do about It?

- Do not use feather, acrylic, chemically treated, or pesticide-treated pillows or comforters.
- Buy only organic cotton bedding and pillows.

Try *www.BioNatural.com* for pure, non-chemically-treated, flame retardant-free cotton pillows and bedding.

Why Is It So Important to Use Natural, Organic Bedding?

- Feather pillows and comforters can exacerbate allergies.

◌ Feather pillows are usually treated chemically to try and stop allergic reactions. If something has to be chemically treated just to make it tolerable for the human body to be near, how safe could it be to sleep on?

◌ Form-fitting pillows are made from a combination of foams and chemical adhesives.

◌ Seven of the top fifteen pesticides used on cotton are classified as, at the least, possible human carcinogens.[9]

◌ It has been reported that "memory foam" pillows are chemically treated and require "airing" before use. You must ask yourself, are these chemicals safe? Can simply "airing out" a chemically-treated mattress or pillow protect against toxic chemicals?

◌ One study found that that the average pillow, be it synthetic or down, contains between four and sixteen different types of fungi, with synthetic pillows having the most. The most common fungus found was Aspergillus fumigatus, which commonly causes asthma attacks and sinusitis.[10]

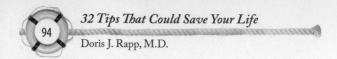

Tip 17: Clothing

Many fabrics used for clothing are treated with chemicals that can be harmful to your health.

What Can You Do about It?

- Buy cotton that wrinkles, silk, ramie, or totally natural fibers.

- Avoid using "wrinkle-free" fabrics.

- Avoid polyester.

- Avoid stain-resistant fabrics, as these may contain Teflon™.

- Beware of pesticides in clothing and children's Halloween costumes.

Why Is Non-Toxic Clothing So Important?

- Fabrics such as permanent-press cotton or other "wrinkle-free" clothing can contain either the chemical DMDHEU (1, 2-Di-methylol-4, 5-dihydroxyethyleneurea) or perfluorinated chemicals (PFCs), including Teflon™.

- DMDHEU contains formaldehyde, which can cause cancer.[11]

- Perfluorinated chemicals cause cancer.[12]

- Polyester also contains formaldehyde.

- Synthetic fabrics can aggravate eczema and cause itching.

- Synthetic leather and vinyl fabrics contain phthalates (plasticizers) that appear to cause an array of health problems. (See Tip #14: Plastic, p.20, and Appendix II, tables 4-7)

Dry Cleaning

About 85% of dry cleaners use chemicals called tri-tetra or perchloroethylenes. This chemical is also found in paint, copiers, spot removers, and degreasers.

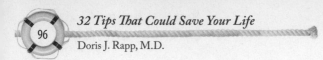

What Can You Do about It?

- ○ If you must wear dry-cleaned clothing, do so as infrequently as possible.

- ○ Wear a cotton t-shirt or other undergarment beneath dry clean clothing to prevent perspiration from getting on the dry-clean-only item, prolonging the time between necessary cleanings.

- ○ Some garments labeled "dry clean only" can be hand washed and laid flat to dry.

- ○ Find a "green" dry cleaner that uses more safe cleaning procedures.

- ○ Never store freshly dry cleaned clothing in your bedroom. Air them out thoroughly outside and then store in a spare bedroom.

- ○ "Wet Cleaning" involves water and detergent milder than what is used in the home combined with professional pressing and finishing equipment. This is an excellent alternative to regular dry cleaning.

○ The EPA has a list of environmentally friendly cleaners available on their website at http://www.epa.gov/epp/pubs/products/cleaning.htm.

Why Is It So Important to Avoid Regular Dry Cleaners?

○ Perchloroethylene, or "perc," is the most common chemical used for dry cleaning. It can cause fatigue, nausea, depression, dizziness, headaches, numbness, confusion, an increased chance of developing lymphomas, and death.[13]

○ It has been reported that you increase your chance of developing cancer by wearing dry-cleaned clothing once per week.[14]

○ Studies among workers in the dry cleaning industry show an increased risk of bladder, esophageal, and cervical cancer; eye, nose, throat, and skin irritation; and reduced fertility.[15]

○ It has been reported that mice develop liver cancer when exposed to the perchloroethylenes used for dry cleaning.[16]

Mothballs

Mothballs generally contain either naphthalene or dichlorobenzene, which are harmful to your health.

What Can You Do about It?

○ Use no mothballs or naphthalene, especially in children's clothing or bedding.

○ Buy some vacuum zip plastic garment storage bags (available at larger chain, grocery, or linen stores).

○ Try essential oils such as cedar, clove, lavender, mint, or orange.

○ Instead of hanging them in a closet, place clothing in drawers with cedar blocks or lavender sachets. The moth-repelling scents work better in smaller spaces.

Why Is It So Important to Avoid Using Mothballs?

- Naphthalene is released directly into the air from factories burning fossil fuels and from mothballs. Air pollution and cigarette smoke are other sources.[17]

- The naphthalene in mothballs is toxic to humans and can cause cataracts, anemia, and problems in respiratory system.[18]

- Naphthalene is absorbed well through the skin. Infants younger than six weeks of age are particularly sensitive to small amounts because their bodies cannot metabolize it. Illness can be severe and recovery time can be prolonged.[18]

- Naphthalene is labeled by the EPA as a possible human carcinogen.[18]

- Short-term exposure causes hemolytic anemia, as well as liver and neurological damage.[18]

- Long-term exposure can cause cataracts and permanent retina damage.[18]

- Naphthalene can cross the placenta in amounts large enough to cause toxicity in unborn babies.[18]

- Anemia has been reported in infants born to mothers who "sniffed" and/or ingested mothballs (naphthalene) during pregnancy. [18]

- The oral absorption of naphthalene is enhanced by solution in oil or ingestion in water rather than in food.

- The chemical was still found in the urine of patients five days after ingesting naphthalene.[18]

- Animal studies show that naphthalene deposits are found in the tissues of the body and detected in the fat, liver, lungs, and heart of pigs. Studies are limited regarding how naphthalene distributes itself in human tissue; however, the anatomy of pigs is very similar to that of humans, and thus these findings raise concern. It has also been found in the liver and milk of dairy cows and in the liver, kidneys, lungs, and fat in laying chickens, as well as in the yolks of their eggs.[19]

○ Dichlorobenzene has been used to replace naphthalene. It causes vomiting in adults, is listed by the EPA as a possible human carcinogen, listed in California's proposition 65, Safe Drinking Water and Toxic Enforcement Act of 1986 as "known to the State to cause cancer," and has caused liver and kidney tumors in animal testing.

Notes

1. Chem-Tox.com. "Child Mattress Emissions Generate Concern." http://www.chem-tox.com/beds/frame-beds.htm (accessed May 9, 2010).

2. Essentia.com. "Hazardous Chemicals Found in Fire-Retardants." www.myessentia.com/research/fire-retardants (accessed May 6, 2010).

3. Strobel.com. "CDC and EPA Proves Flameproof Mattress Toxic." http://www.strobel.com/cdc__epa_proves_flameproof_matt.htm (accessed May 6, 2010).

4. Agency for Toxic Substances and Disease Registry. "Toxicological Profile for Antimony Compounds." 1992. http://www.atsdr.cdc.gov/toxprofiles/tp23.pdf.

5. Environmental Protection Agency. "Antimony (CASRN 7440-36-0)." 2010. http://www.epa.gov/iris/subst/0006.htm

6. Sprott, Jim. "Look at Cots to Isolate Possible Cause of SIDS." 1995. http://www.pnc.com.au/~cafmr/sprott/sids-gas.html (accessed May 6, 2010).

7. MyparenTime.com. "SIDS Part IV: How much Do We Really Know About This Mysterious Killer of Babies?." www.myparentime.com/articles/article103d.shtml (accessed May 6, 2010).

8 MyparenTime.com. "SIDS Part IV: How much Do We Really Know About This Mysterious Killer of Babies?." www.myparentime.com/articles/article103d.shtml (accessed May 6, 2010).

9. Organic Consumers Assocation. "Fact Sheet on U.S. Cotton Subsidies and Cotton Production." www.organicconsumers.org/clothes/224subsidies.cfm (accessed May 6, 2010).

10. Science Daily.com. "Pillows: A Hotbed of Fungus Spores." 2005. www.sciencedaily.com/releases/2005/10/051015093046. html (accessed May 6, 2010).

11. Thomason, Spencer. "Optimization of Ionic Crosslinking." PhD diss., North Carolina University, 2006. http://www.lib.ncsu. edu/theses/available/etd-05042006-142014/unrestricted/etd.pdf.

12. Pollution In People.Org. "Perfluorinated Compounds: Stain Protecters Leave an Indelible Mark." http://pollutioninpeople. org/toxics/pfcs (accessed May 7, 2010).

13 National Library of Medicine ToxNet. "Tetrachloroethylene." http://toxnet.nlm.nih.gov/cgi-bin/sis/ search/f?./temp/~fTHReL:1 (accessed May 7, 2010).

14. Dakss, Brian. "Cancer Danger from Dry Cleaning?" Tracy Smith Explores Possible Risk of Commonly Used Chemical Called "PERC". 2007. www.cbsnews.com/stories/2007/02/23/ earlyshow/contributors/tracysmith/main/2507444.shtml (accessed May 7, 2010).

15. NTP. "11th Report On Carcinogens for Tetrachloroethylene." 2005. http://ntp.niehs.nih.gov/ntp/roc/ eleventh/profiles/s169tetr.pdf.

16. Halogenated Solvents Industry Alliance, Inc. "Perchloroethylene White Paper." 2008. www.hsia.org/white_ papers/perc%20wp%202008.htm.

17. Agency for Toxic Substances and Disease Registry. "Naphthalene ToxFAQs." 2005. http://www.atsdr.cdc.gov/ tfacts67.pdf.

18. Environmental Protection Agency. "Health Effects Support Document for Naphthalene." 2003. http://www.epa.gov/ safewater/ccl/pdfs/reg_determine1/support_cc1_naphthalene_ healtheffects.pdf.

19. Eisele, GR. "Naphthalene Distribution in Tissues of Laying Pullets, Swine and Dairy Cattle." *Bulletin of Environmental*

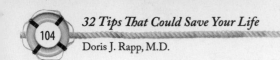

Contamination and Toxicology 34 (1985): 549-556, http://www.
springerlink.com/content/q17571119w46l639/?p=4f388642a3384
b4ca7dd75bfa6a003fa&pi=79.

Chapter 5

The Bathroom

Tip 18: Dental Care

Most dental devices, fillings, and care products contain harmful ingredients. While the best way to avoid them is to take excellent care of your teeth and prevent cavities and dental problems altogether, this is not always possible for everyone.

What Can You Do about It?

- Allow only ceramic/porcelain, never composite, mercury, or metal fillings. Gold fillings tend to be mixed with toxic metals as well.

- Choose dental appliances such as retainers, aligners, braces, and dentures carefully.

- Have any existing amalgam (mercury) fillings removed and replaced with safer materials.

- Avoid root canals. They are pockets for infection that cause symptoms as time passes.

- Most brands of mouthwash contain saccharin or aspartame. Choose natural brands that are naturally sweetened.

Why Is Safer Dental Care So Important?

- Mercury in metal filling material can slowly be released from the fillings and can poison the body over time. Mercury toxicity can cause allergies, rheumatoid arthritis, memory loss, multiple sclerosis, epilepsy, vision problems, immune suppression, mental confusion, migraine headaches, and depression. It can also hinder the absorption of nutrients in the body. I personally believe that it contributes to the current autism epidemic.[1]

○ Composite fillings, adhesive used to attach braces, dentures, and other dental devices such as some retainers and aligners can contain bisphenol-A as a hardener. As previously mentioned in Tip #7: Plastic, Bisphenol-A can cause a multitude of health problems and should be avoided if at all possible.

○ It is best to check on brands of retainers and aligners that report they do not contain BPA or phthalates.

○ Some dental patients who have their mercury amalgam fillings removed and replaced with porcelain can experience a total disappearance of unexplained health issues such as depression, arthritis, and heart and blood pressure problems. For others, however, the experience does not appear to improve their health. It is an expensive gamble. You might experience a miracle, but even if you don't, it is better to have this major source of toxic metals removed. This is especially true for women who want to have children

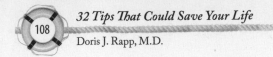

because the mercury in the mouth can cross the placenta and pass into the unborn child.[2] A biological dentist, who knows how to properly remove this type of filling without releasing more mercury into your system during the process, is certainly preferred.

Toothpaste:

Most regular toothpastes contain fluoride, sodium lauryl sulfate, triclosan and hydrated silica.

What Can You Do about It?

- Use organic, non-fluoridated toothpaste.
- Use only organic toothpaste from health food stores.
- Read Dr. Robert Bernardini's book, *The Truth About Children's Health*.

Why Is It So Important to Be Careful with Toothpaste Choices?

- A pea-sized amount of fluoridated toothpaste has been reported to be unsafe if swallowed by a seven-year-old.[3]

- Fluoride is the main ingredient in some insecticides.[4]

- A Harvard graduate student found five times more bone cancer in young males using fluoride.[5]

- An overabundance of fluoride in the body can lead to fluorosis, a condition afflicting many people in rural India where clean, purified drinking water is difficult to obtain. This condition has spread among urban residents, being ingested mainly through food. Fluorosis can cause back and joint pain, low energy levels and fatigue along with brittle, discolored teeth that are often very yellow or brown all over or in lines across the teeth (bleaching or whitening only helps in some cases). The National

Health and Nutrition Examination Survey showed that levels of fluorosis in U.S. children rose from 22.8% in 1986-1987 to 32% in 2002 and then to 41% in 2007.[6]

- A 1997 study showed that drinking water with 2 ppm (parts per million) of fluoride, one-half of the US EPA's recommended safe level, caused liver and kidney disturbances in children.[7]

- Fluoride has been linked to ADHD at 100 ppm (parts per million). Some toothpastes can contain up to 1500 ppm.[8,9]

- Many toothpastes contain sodium lauryl sulfate, triclosan, and hydrated silica. All of these can be a concern.

- Sodium lauryl sulfate (SLS) is used in lab testing to intentionally irritate the skin.

- Triclosan is a pesticide.

- Hydrated silica is an abrasive and is added to toothpaste to help remove plaque, but what else is it removing? It is also an ingredient used in some paints and varnishes. When it is dehydrated, it is known as silica gel. Packets of silica gel are often placed in shoes and other packages to control humidity and bear a label warning that it is not for consumption.

An Example of a Patient with Fluoride Sensitivity:

<u>Marcia</u>

History:

- ✿ Marcia had classic allergies and chemical sensitivities. Fluoride was a major part of her medical problems.

- ✿ When Marcia was eight years old, the family moved to another town, and she was placed on fluoride tablets. In a few weeks, she was extremely depressed and cried all the time.

- ✿ She could not attend school and had no desire to learn.

- She also had fatigue, difficulty concentrating, muscle aches, headaches, and problems walking.

- She saw over twenty doctors and specialists, and no one could figure out the change in her behavior. Her mother told the doctors that she thought it was the fluoride, but she was assured that could not be the cause.

- Marcia was placed in a psychiatric hospital for children, and they suggested that she stay there for an indefinite period because counseling was not effective, and Marcia continued to be very depressed.

- Some doctors tried to blame the parents even though there was no evidence to support that consideration.

Treatment:

- When Marcia came to our office, she drew pictures of animals until we administered several drops of a solution made from dissolved fluoride tablets.

- Shortly thereafter, she became very sad and drew tears on her pictures of the dogs. She was treated with the correct dilution of fluoride, and in a few minutes, she was no longer sad and changed her pictures to happy faces.

- Once she was treated, her I.Q. increased from 57 to 125 over a period of several months.

- She became a bubbly, happy, and energetic child who danced and lived a normal, active life.

- Her treatment consisted of making the home more allergy-free and taking nutrients and allergy extract treatment for foods, dust, molds, and pollen. Most importantly, however, she no longer had any contact with fluoride. To see the video of this fluoride reaction, go to www.drrapp. com.

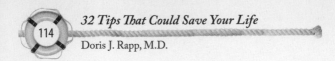

Tip 19: Personal Body Products

Lotions, creams, lipstick, moisturizers, and other personal products can contain toxic and cancer-causing ingredients.

What Can You Do about It?

- Beware of any personal products containing one or more the following:
  - Lauryl sulfate
  - DEA cocamide
  - Quaternium 15
  - Propylene glycol (antifreeze)
  - Talc
- Use no regular fingernail polish and remover. They're possibly safer if purchased from health food stores.
- Buy body products at health stores, and use organic coconut or jojoba oil as a moisturizer.

○ Watch your perfumes. They do not have to tell what is in their scents because it is a trade secret. Some can contain numerous causes of cancer, but they are not required to tell those who use the products. If you become sick after using your perfume—some might have an elevated pulse or problems breathing—consider that something in the perfumes might be bothering you. Long term effects such as cancer are difficult to prove.

○ Look for safe, organic insect repellent for the skin. There are reports that those listed below may be "safer" alternatives:[10]

   ○ Bite Blocker

   ○ All Terrain Herbal Armor (5 oils to deter bites)

○ Avoid Deet in insect repellents. It can be toxic on sunburns or in high concentrations in children.

○ Read Samuel S. Epstein's *Unreasonable Risk* and *Cancer Gate* (1-800-638-7819)

Why Is Using Caution with Personal Body Products So Important?

- Many cosmetic manufacturers do not have to reveal toxins or cancer-causing substances in their products because it is a "trade secret."

- Lauryl Sulfate is reported to cause irritation after extended exposure.

- DEA cocamide can cause cancer.

- Quaternium 15 is a formaldehyde releaser, which is a chemical that is a carcinogen.[11]

- Propylene glycol is used as a "less toxic" antifreeze and as the insecticide in traps used to capture and kill ground beetles. It is also the main ingredient in deodorant sticks.

- Several studies have established preliminary links between talc and lung damage, as well as with skin and ovarian cancer.[12]

- Most beauty products contain paraben, which is linked to breast cancer over time. Parabens accumulate in the fatty tissues of the body. These chemicals mimic estrogen and may be a reason for why young women are experiencing infertility and why girls are entering puberty earlier now than in the past.

○ Nail polish often contains phthalates, which are reported to cause the male offspring of rats to become more feminine and possibly to have abnormal reproductive organs, while the female offspring have more miscarriages.

A Teacher with Multiple Sensitivities to Perfumes and Hair Sprays

Nancy

History:

○ For about eight years, Nancy had progressively more and more fatigue and muscle aches.

○ She had drastic mood swings and excessive crying associated with irritability.

- She had numb fingers and skin, head-aches, dizziness, muscle spasms, and problems concentrating.

- Nancy saw many doctors without relief or answers. She was particularly bad in the spring. At times, she was too tired to get out of bed, shower, or even eat. It took twenty minutes to crawl from her bedroom to the nearby bathroom.

Treatment:

- After Provocation/Neutralization testing, she improved dramatically.

- She also took nutrients, exercised, and took other measures to detoxify her body.

- In time, she could tolerate exposures to many of the items that had previously rendered her unable to function normally.

- She continues to be cautious so that she is not overwhelmed and incapacitated by her many sensitivities.

Triggers and Symptoms:

- Nancy became sensitive if she was exposed to mold, dust, perfume, and especially to phenol, which are commonly found in school and home disinfectants.

- The smell of perfume could make her so confused that she couldn't think or remember. At times she would laugh uncontrollably and develop tics and twitches.

- During a television appearance with Dr. Rapp, Nancy was speaking normally when another guest, who smelled of hair spray and perfume, came on stage and sat down next to her. In seconds, Nancy's voice became hoarse, and she could barely breathe. She was quickly taken outside, and in a few minutes she felt fine again. To see the video of this fluoride reaction, go to www.drrapp.com.

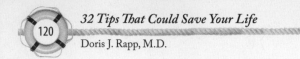
Tip 20: Female Products

Some sanitary products are bleached white
with toxic chemicals. In addition, many creams
made for female use should be avoided because
of the irritants they contain.

What Can You Do about It?

- Use only natural sanitary products.

- Try Natracare feminine products. They
  are totally organic feminine care products that are not bleached with dioxin.
  They are safer because of how they are
  made. They can be purchased at many
  natural food and chain stores, as well as
  online. Visit *www.NatraCare.com*.

- Do not use any estrogen or yeast
  infection cream that contains propylene
  glycol. Choose products that do not
  contain this chemical or request that a
  compounding pharmacy create a
  propylene-glycol-free cream for you.

Why are Safer Sanitary Products So Important?

- Some sanitary pads, tampons, and liners are bleached with dioxin, which may be related to the rise in endometriosis.

  - Some dioxin derivatives are directly linked with an increase in the likelihood of developing cancer.[13]

  - Agent Orange, used in the Vietnam War, contained dioxin. Men and dogs exposed to it were found to have increased testicular cancer.[14]

- A study at the University of Maryland School of Medicine found that dioxin causes vaginal defects in unborn rats. A web of tissue forms that partially obstructs the vaginal opening and may impair the rat's reproductive ability.

- Propylene glycol is added to many estrogen and yeast infection creams as a moisturizer, but sometimes it can cause extreme vaginal burning and irritation.

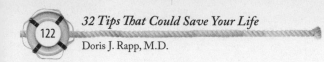
Tip 21: Hair Color and Perms

Some regular hair dyes and permanent wave solutions contain extremely hazardous chemicals that can damage your hair and body.

What Can You Do about It?

- Avoid regular hair dyes, and use all-natural dyes instead.

- Choose safer hair dyes and permanent wave solutions available at health food stores.

- Use lemon juice to lighten and brighten blonde hair or to add blonde highlights.

- Henna is also a natural way to produce red shades. Boxed henna hair color is available at many health food stores and some chain grocery and drug stores.

- Instead of perming, use overnight rollers to get your curls. You will avoid harmful perm chemicals, which is better for your health and your hair.

⬭ Aubrey Organics makes all-natural hair color. Visit *www. Aubrey-organics.com* Many all natural hair care products and dyes are available at health food stores.

Why Is It So Important to Use Safer Hair Dyes?

⬭ Some regular hair dyes can cause cancer.

⬭ Some regular hair dyes contain ammonia. This can be corrosive to human tissue.

  ⚬ It can cause skin and eye irritation in low concentrations, and skin burns, permanent eye damage, or even blindness in higher concentrations such as those found in commercial/industrial cleaners.

  ⚬ When inhaled, ammonia can cause immediate feelings of burning in the nose, throat, and respiratory tract. It damages the airway, which can result in breathing problems.

⬭ The FDA requires that hair dye boxes carry a warning stating that blindness can occur after the use of hair dye on eyebrows or eyelashes.

- Accidentally ingesting permanent hair wave solutions, which contain bromate, can cause vomiting, stomach pain, diarrhea, low blood pressure, loss of reflexes, anemia, kidney problems, and hearing loss. Death can occur as a result of the kidney damage if it is not immediately treated.

- The EPA considers bromate to be a probable human carcinogen.

Notes

1. Huggins, HA, Levy, TE. *Uninformed Consent: The Hidden Dangers In Dental Care*. Newburyport: Hampton Roads Publishing Company, Inc., 1999.

2. Ask, K., A. Akesson, M. Berglund, and M. Vahter. "Inorganic Mercury and Methylmercury in Placentas of Swedish Women." *Environmental Health Perspectives*. 110, no. 5 (2002): 523-526.

3. Warning on toothpaste label.

4. Metcalf, R.L. "Fluorine-Containing Insecticides." in *Introduction to Chapter 7, Handbook of Experimental Pharmacology*. Springer, Berlin-Heidelber-New York, 1966.

5. Bassin, E. B., D. Wypij, R. B. Davis, M. A. Mittleman. "Age-specific fluoride exposure in drinking water and osteosarcoma (United States)." *Cancer Causes Control* 17 (2006): 421-428.

6. Beltran-Aguilar ED, Griffin SO, Lockwood SA. "Prevalence and trends in enamel fluorosis in the United States from the 1930s to the 1980s." *Journal of the American Dental Association* 133 (2002): 157-165.

7. Committee on Fluoride in Drinking Water, National Research Council. "Fluoride in Drinking Water: A Scientific Review of EPA's Standards." National Academies Press. 2006. http://books.nap.edu/openbook.php?record_id=11571&page=R1#.

8. Mullenix, Patricia, et al. "Neurotoxicity of sodium fluoride in rats." *Neurotoxicology and Teratology* 17 (1995): 69-177.

9. Hellwig, Elmar, et al. "Remineralization of initial carious lesions in deciduous enamel after application of dentifrices of different fluoride concentrations." *Clinical Oral*

Investigations (June 2009), http://www.springerlink.com/content/c708664nt7462r75/.

10. Sezben, Naomi. "Non-Toxic Insect Repellants: A Safer Alternative to Bug Sprays." http://natural-products.suite101.com/article.cfm/nontoxic_insect_repellents (accessed May 4, 2010).

11. De Groot, Anton C, et al. "Formaldehyde releasers: relationship to to formaldehyde contact allergy. Contact allergy to formaldehyde and inventory of formaldehyde-releasers." *Contact Dermatitis* 61 (2009): 63-85.

12. Powell, Ashley. "Does Talc Baby Powder Cause Lung Disease, Tumors, Ovarian Cancer, Immune Problems, and Pneumonia?." *American Chronicle* (June 2009), www.americanchronicle.com.

13. Schecter, Arnold and James R. Olsen. "Cancer risk assessment using blood dioxin levels and daily TEQ intake levels in general populations of industrial and non-industrial countries." *Chemosphere* 34 (1997):1569-1577.

14. Chamie, Karim, et. al. "Agent Orange exposure, Viet Nam war veterans, and the risk of prostate cancer." *Cancer* 113 (2008):1-7.

Chapter 6

Caring for Your Child

Tip 22: Diapering

Some disposable infant diapers can contain harmful chemicals and should be avoided. Disposable baby wipes can contain skin irritants.

What Can You Do about It?

- ✪ It is best to use a diaper service and natural, unbleached cotton diapers. Do not, however, use the plastic covers that are often used with cloth diapers. Doing this nullifies the benefits of cloth diapers. There are safer cloth covers available that appear to be effective.

- ✪ Tushies brand diapers are available at health stores. They are the only disposable diaper made with cotton and do not contain the gel filling used by other "green" and organic disposables that are available at health food stores.

🔹 To prevent skin irritation, choose baby wipes that are fragrance-free and do not contain propylene glycol.

Why are Safer Diapers and Wipes So Important?

🔹 Many disposable diapers contain plastic in the form of bisphenol A (BPA), which is reported to make male infants more effeminate.[1]

🔹 Scented baby wipes contain artificial fragrances, known sources of phthalates, which studies link with smaller genitals and incompletely descended testicles in human males.[2]

🔹 Doctors at the University of Kiel in Germany have raised concerns about the correlation between disposable, plastic lined diapers and rising male infertility. Disposable diapers with plastic linings have been found to maintain boys' testicles at higher than normal temperatures. This has been linked to reduced sperm counts due to the rise in temperature of the genitals.[3]

- Many brands of baby wipes contain propylene glycol, which is linked to rashes, deafness, kidney damage, and liver problems. This chemical is reported to cause vaginal burning and irritation in adult women when used in vaginal creams.

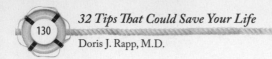

Tip 23:
Pregnancy and Chemicals

PCBs (polychlorinated biphenyls) and other chemicals pass through the placenta into the unborn. Some exposures have been known to cause devastating birth defects. These chemicals have also been found in breast milk.[4]

What Can You Do about It?

- Stay as far away as possible from pesticide-treated areas.

- Do not eat pesticide-laden food or any fish from the Great Lakes. Try to eat only organic foods.

- If your job requires you to be in contact with any chemicals or pesticides, insist that other tasks be given to you for the duration of your pregnancy.

Why Is It So Important to Avoid Chemical Exposure During Pregnancy?

- In 2004, a group of farm workers were reportedly directed to work with gloves but without adequate protective equipment in heavily pesticide-treated fields. Up to eighteen pesticides were applied at triple the legal frequency, even while workers were in the fields. Babies born to three of the women working under these conditions had birth defects. One baby was born without arms or legs and with spinal and lung defects.[5] The parents of the children sued the company, and it was determined that the heavy exposure to the many pesticides were responsible for the children's deformities.[6]

- Babies with higher concentrations of PCBs in their umbilical cord blood tend to have

  - lower birth weight,

  - smaller than normal head size,

  - developmental delays.[7]

○ Studies have shown that children of mothers who were exposed to PCBs while pregnant developed a number of permanent physical and neurological problems, including

　○ movement, mental, and behavioral problems;

　○ increased activity levels;

　○ slowed thought processing and "less bright" appearance;

　○ lower reaction times and greater hyperactivity;

　○ compromised nervous systems;

　○ reductions in thyroid hormone levels. If the thyroid gland does not function well before birth and throughout the first two months after birth, a child's brain will not develop normally. There is a similarity in the type of nervous system damage noted in thyroid disorders and those noted after PCB and dioxin exposure;

- boys had smaller penises and were more feminine at play;

- PCB's appear to cause girls to be more masculine at play. In contrast, other chemicals can make girls more feminine.[7]

- There are an estimated 2,800 chemicals in the Great Lakes water. The more PCBs in a lake, the more found in the fish. If pregnant women eat these fish, their babies tend to be twitchier, have poorer balance, weaker reflexes, developmental delays, smaller heads, and lower IQs.

- Infants with higher levels of PCBs were found to have more learning difficulties as they grew up. By four years of age, those exposed to the highest PCB levels had the lowest verbal and memory test scores.

- One study showed that boys exposed in-utero have smaller penises.

- Numerous studies have also confirmed similar significant genital changes in aquatic and wild animals.[7]

○ Organophosphates pose a high risk for pregnant women. These include Bisphenol-A and phthalates. They are derived from World War II nerve agents and are highly toxic. Even at low levels, organophosphates can be toxic to the developing brain, and studies show that they can affect brain and reproductive development in unborn animals. While most pesticides categorized as organophosphates have been banned for household use, they are still permitted for commercial use, including in fumigation for mosquitoes.[8] Malathion, a common toxic organophosphate, is still allowed for use as an industrial and household insecticide. In the US, approximately 15 million pounds of malathion are used each year by the government, as well as by businesses and homeowners.[9]

○ It is most discouraging that some communities continue to use malathion, as well as other toxic chemicals, to control mosquitoes when safer measures are known and readily available. Refer to my book *Our Toxic World, A Wake Up Call*. 1-800-787-8780.

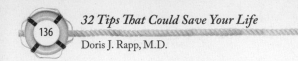
Tip 24: Vaccinations

When the recommendations of the U.S. government for immunizations are followed, a five-year-old American child will have received more than 30 doses of various vaccines, many containing mercury, formaldehyde, and aluminum.

What Can You Do about It?

○ Become informed about the vaccine and the illness it prevents before consenting to having it. Are the remedies for the illness safer than the vaccine that prevents it? Decide whether this immunization is right for you, and always avoid any unnecessary vaccines.

○ Ask your doctor to explain to you all of the risks and benefits of each immunization. Ask why each vaccine is recommended and whether it is a legal requirement or simply a recommendation. You have a right to know what is going into your body or your child's body. If your doctor does not have the time to adequately answer your questions about vaccinations, find a new doctor.

- Do not receive vaccinations when sick. If your child is ill and due for shots, call and reschedule, giving the child time to fully recover before the immunization.

- If you decide on vaccinations for your children, schedule them one at a time. Physicians often want to do several in one visit, but this means injecting more mercury into your child. Some believe this can increase the risk for an adverse reaction.

- Most daycare centers and schools require immunizations for enrollment; however, every state has exemptions. Every immunization law grants exemptions for medical reasons. All but two U.S. states allow religious exemptions. Some also allow for philosophical exemptions, and this trend is becoming more popular. NMA Media Press publishes *Say No to Vaccines* by Dr.

Sherri Tenpenny, and New Atlantean Press publishes a booklet entitled *How to Legally Avoid Vaccines in All 50 States*.

○ For self-treating the flu:

 ○ Oscillococcinum, available at drugstores and health food stores, is one homeopathic remedy that appears to be helpful.

 ○ Vitamin D appears to be helpful.

 ○ Dr. Joseph Mercola claims that he has not received a flu shot in twenty years, and has not had the flu even once. He attributes this good health to exercise, getting adequate sleep, addressing his emotional stresses, washing his hands (but not excessively), and maintaining a diet that includes abstaining from sugar, eating garlic regularly and consuming a high-quality krill oil daily. (Dr. Joseph Mercola, 10/21/2008, *Avoid Flu Shots With the One Vitamin that Will Stop Flu in Its Tracks*)

Why is it So Important to Avoid Some Vaccines?

- Vaccines in general can contain mercury, formaldehyde, and aluminum.

  - Mercury levels in immunizations are believed by many parents and some physicians to be a cause of autism.[10]

  - Mercury can cause damage to the brain, kidney, and lungs.[11]

  - Formaldehyde is a human carcinogen.

  - Aluminum has been linked to Alzheimer's disease.[12]

- Vaccines can sometimes trigger Guillain-Barre Syndrome (GBS), a rare but potentially devastating autoimmune disorder that can cause paralysis.[13]

- Delaying infant vaccinations by two months appears to dramatically reduce the risk of childhood asthma.[14]

- Flu shots:

  - Fifty-one studies of 250,000 children

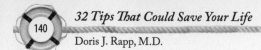

show that flu vaccines are only as effective as a placebo.[15]

○ It is reported that flu shots, which are frequently urged for those younger than five years old, have been shown to be ineffective and to sometimes cause flu-like symptoms. Nasal spray forms of the flu vaccine do contain a live flu virus that is weakened." [16]

○ Vaccines do not protect the elderly against pneumonia. Even though 15% were vaccinated in 1960 and 65% now, the number of deaths is the same. It appears to be of no or little benefit.[17]

○ Human Papillomavirus Vaccines:

○ The human immune system in older women, who are the ones most likely to develop this problem, is usually strong enough to clear up HPV infection on its own and does so in most women. The CDC admits to this fact on their website; however, they still recommend that it be given to young girls. Long-term studies showing the length of time the vaccine lasts are still needed. The vaccine protects against the major four, out of 140 strains of the viruses that cause HPV.

- Nine thousand "adverse events," including the deaths of eighteen girls and young women, ten spontaneous abortions, six cases of Guillain-Barre Syndrome; and twenty-seven events considered to be "life-threatening" have been reported as adverse effects from Gardasil.[18]

- Gardasil contains Polysorbate-80, which has been linked to infertility in mice.[19]

Notes

1. "Scientists Link Infertility and Testicular Cancer to Disposable Diapers." http://www.babyloveproducts.com/data/maleinfertility.html (accessed on June 6, 2010).

2. Swan, SH, KM Main, F Liu, SL Stewart, RL Kruse, AM Calafat, CS Mao, JB Redmon, CL Ternand, S Sullivan, JL Teague, EZ Drobnis, BS Carter, D Kelly, TM Simmons, C Wang, L Lumbreras, S Villanueva, M Diaz-Romero, MB Lomeli, E Otero-Salazar, C Hobel, B Brock, C Kwong, A Muehlen, A Sparks, A Wolk, J Whitham, M Hatterman-Zogg, M Maifield and The Study for Future Families Research Group. "Decrease in Anogenital Distance Among Male Infants with Prenatal Phthalate Exposure." *Environmental Health Perspectives* 113 (2005): 1056-1061, http://www.ourstolenfuture.org/NewScience/oncompounds/phthalates/2005/2005-0527swanetal.htm.

3. Dada, R, NP Gupta and K Kucheria. "Spermatogenic arrest in men with testicular hyperthermia." *Teratogenesis, Carcinogenesis, and Mutagenesis* S1 (2003): 235-43, http://www3.interscience.wiley.com/journal/103020520/abstract?CRETRY=1&SRETRY=0.

4. Kostyniak, P.J., C. Stinson, H.B. Greizerstein, J. Vena, G. Buck, P. Mendola,. "Relation of Lake Ontario Fish Consumption, Lifetime Lactation, and Parity to Breast Milk Polychlorobiphenyl and Pesticide Concentrations." *Environmental Research Section* A 80, no 2 pt. 2 (1999): S166-S174.

5. Lantigua, John. "Pesticides the Root Cause of Birth Defects in Farmworkers," *Palm Beach Post*, March 13, 2005. http://www.organicconsumers.org/OFGU/birthdefects031405.cfm.

6. Bishop, Katy. "Parents of Child Born Without Limbs Settle With Tomato Grower," *Naples News*, March 24, 2008. http://

www.naplesnews.com/news/2008/mar/24/parents-child-born-without-limbs-settle-tomato-gro/.

7. "PCB Baby Studies, Parts 1, 2 and 3." Fox River Watch. http://www.foxriverwatch.com/baby_studies_pcbs_1.html, http://www.foxriverwatch.com/baby_studies_pcbs_2.html, http://www.foxriverwatch.com/baby_studies_pcbs_3.html.

8. Mehl, Anna, Tore M. Schanke, Bjorn A. Johnsen and Frode Fonnum "The effect of trichlorfon and other organophosphates on prenatal brain development in the guinea pig." *Neurochemical Research* 19, no. 5 (May 1994).

9. "Reregistration Eligibility Decision (RED) for Malathion." US EPA. http://www.epa.gov/oppsrrd1/REDs/malathion_red.pdf.

10. http://www.wnd.com/?pageId=35079.

11. Countera , S. Allen, and Leo H. Buchananb "Mercury exposure in children: a review." *Toxicology and Applied Pharmacology* 198 (2004) 209–230.

12. Klatzo. I. et al. "Experimental production of neurofibrillary degeneration: I. Light microscopic observations." *Journal of Neuropathology & Experimental Neurology* 24 (1965):187-199.

13. Sejvar J, Y. Mikaeloff, F. DeStefano. "Vaccines and Guillain-Barré syndrome." *Drug Safety.* 32, no. 4 (2009): 309-23, http://www.ncbi.nlm.nih.gov/pubmed/19388722.

14. McDonald KL, S.I. Huq, L. M. Lix, A. B. Becker, A. L. Kozyrskyj. "Delay in diphtheria, pertussis, tetanus vaccination is associated with a reduced risk of childhood asthma." *Journal of Allergy and Clinical Immunology.* 121, no. 3 (2008): 626-31, http://www.ncbi.nlm.nih.gov/pubmed/18207561.

15. "The Toddler Debate." *The Washington Post.* Tuesday, January 31, 2006 http://www.washingtonpost.com/wpdyn/content/article/2006/01/30/AR2006013001253.html.

16. Dr. Mercola. "Flu Vaccine Exposed." http://articles.mercola.

com/sites/articles/archive/2009/09/26/Flu-Vaccine-Exposed.aspx
(accessed on June 29, 2010)

17. Archives of Internal Medicine. February 12, 2005.

18. "A Judicial Watch Special Report: Examining the FDA's
HPV Vaccine Records - Detailing the Approval Process,
Side-Effects, Safety Concerns and Marketing Practices
of a Large-Scale Public Health Experiment." June 30,
2008. http://www.judicialwatch.org/documents/2008/
JWReportFDAhpvVaccineRecords.pdf.

19. Gajdová M, J. Jakubovsky, J. Války. "Delayed effects of
neonatal exposure to Tween 80 on female reproductive organs
in rats." *Food and Chemical Toxicology* 31, no. 3 (1993): 183-90,
http://www.ncbi.nlm.nih.gov/pubmed/8473002.

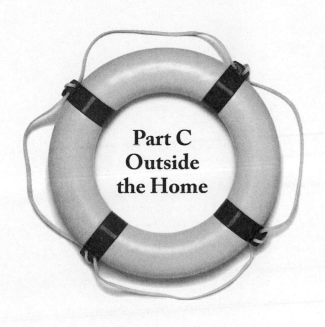

**Part C
Outside
the Home**

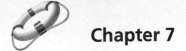

Chapter 7

School, Work, and Play

Tip 25: Reading Materials

Paper found in books, magazines, and newspapers are often treated with several chemicals to enhance their physical quality and attract consumers to certain products.

What Can You Do about It?

- Avoid smelly, shiny white paper in certain books or newspapers (especially the colored sectors). Notice if they cause any symptoms.

- Dry pages with a hair dryer in a well ventilated area and be careful not to breathe in any fumes.

- Pay attention to how you feel after contact with different types of paper. You may feel sleepy, asthmatic, congested, or have trouble concentrating. Does the paper smell? Has ink transferred to your fingers? Do symptoms occur with all shiny prints or just newsprint, certain books, etc.?

Why is it So Important to Choose Reading Materials Carefully?

- The inks or dyes and chemicals in paper can cause illness in some people.

- Styrene, butadiene, and polyethylene are chemicals used to make paper stronger, enhance the way it absorbs colors, and protect the ink from running.

  - Human studies have shown that styrene causes impaired vision, increased reaction times, and decreased memory and concentration.[1]

  - The EPA labels butadiene as carcinogenic to humans.

○ Polyethylene is not biodegradable and ends up deposited in landfills and oceans, where it will take centuries to break down.[2]

○ Many paper mills use chlorine bleach to whiten paper products, creating dioxin. Some dioxin derivatives have repeatedly been reported to increase human chances of developing cancer.[3]

A Child Sensitive to Many Paper Products

Alice:

History:

Alice was sensitive to an array of chemicals, as you may remember from reading about her earlier in the book. In addition to her other sensitivities, Alice developed symptoms from ditto papers, duplicating fluid, fresh newsprint, and paper in new books.

Triggers and Symptoms:

- Duplicating Fluid: One hour after exposure to duplicating fluid, she became giddy, rolled on the floor, began to cough, talked like a baby, and laughed for no apparent reason.

- Ditto Copies: A dry piece of ditto paper caused Alice to change from calm and happy to tired and angry. She could not draw as well as previously and began to scribble. Typical of patients with chemical sensitivities, she could easily smell chemicals on paper even though no odor was apparent to most people.

Treatment:

Alice was treated with Provocation/Neutralization for many of her allergies and sensitivities and she became better quickly. Her reactions could be stopped within ten minutes after receiving the correct environmental allergy extract therapy. To see the video of her reactions, go to www.drrapp.com.

Tip 26: Art Materials

Paints, markers, pens, highlighters, clay, adhesives, and any other art supply you can think of can contain toxic ingredients. Although hazardous products must bear a warning label noting that they contain harmful ingredients and require caution, the U.S. government does not require the manufacturers to list actual ingredients on art supplies.

What Can You Do about It?

- Avoid chemical marking pens, smelly or food odor crayons, and the unpleasant chemical aroma of correction fluid.

- Use only non-toxic art supplies, i.e., paints, crayons, markers, etc.

- The Art & Creative Materials Institute, Inc., (ACMI) is responsible for federally mandated warning labels on hazardous materials. For a list of approved art supplies, visit *www.ACMInet.org*.

- Try the following recipes for non-toxic children's art supplies:

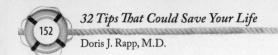
Non-toxic, Edible Art Supply Recipes

While these recipes are nontoxic, they may cause a reaction in children who are sensitive to certain ingredients, such as gluten or food dyes. As an alternative, rice, corn, or chickpea flour can be substituted for wheat flour and natural colorings such as vegetable juices can replace the colorings used in the recipe.

○ Homemade Edible Finger paints

Ingredients:

2 cups flour

2 packets unsweetened Kool-Aid/ other colored, powdered drink mix, or one package of colored gelatin mix.

1/2 cup salt

3 cups boiling water

3 Tbsp vegetable oil

Mix dry ingredients and then add liquid. Mix until smooth.

○ Edible Play-Dough

Ingredients:

1 cup flour

1/2 cup salt

1 cup water

1 tablespoon oil

2 teaspoons Cream of Tartar

1 (3-1/2 oz.) package unsweetened, colored gelatin mix or unsweetened powdered drink mix such as Kool-Aid

Mix dry ingredients.

Heat water over medium heat and add dry ingredients, stirring constantly until thick like mashed potatoes. Remove from heat, and cool until you can comfortably knead on a lightly floured surface until it becomes smooth and is no longer sticky.

Why Are Safe, Non-toxic Art Materials So Important?

- Some clays contain aluminum, which has been linked to Alzheimer's.

- Harmful Ingredients Found in Adhesives/Glues:

  - Acrylonitrile, benzene, and formaldehyde are labeled as human carcinogens.

  - Acrylonitrile is highly flammable and toxic. The burning material releases fumes of hydrogen cyanide and oxides of nitrogen.

  - Butanone causes irritation of the nose, throat, skin, and eyes. If breathed along with other chemicals that damage health, it can increase the amount of harm that occurs.

  - Repeated exposure to cyanoacrylate can result in flu-like symptoms, skin irritation, asthma, and allergic skin reactions.

- Markers can contain harmful solvents such as xylene, toluene, ketone, and alcohol. Crayons marketed for children and labeled non-toxic do not contain these; however, crayons and markers made for adult use may contain toxins.

- Human studies with xylene show neurological impairment and possible developmental effects, as well as an increased incidence of fetuses with retarded bone development or extra ribs.[3]

- Exposure to toluene can cause a host of health effects, including headache, dizziness, and throat, respiratory, and eye irritation. Exposure in pregnant women has been linked to miscarriage, as well as birth defects, attention deficits, and skeletal abnormalities in the unborn child.[5]

- Many of the numerous harmful ingredients in paint can trigger asthma attacks, eye irritation, respiratory problems, nausea, and dizziness.

Prolonged exposure to paint fumes
has been linked to kidney and liver
disease and cancer.[6] Exposure to paint
stripping chemical fumes has been
linked to cancer.[7]

Notes

1. Pollution Prevention and Toxics (November 1994), OPPT
"Chemical Fact Sheets, Styrene Fact Sheet (CAS No. 100-42-5)."
United States Environmental Protection Agency. http://www.epa.
gov/chemfact/styre-fs.txt.

2. "Dioxin: A serious concern for Maine." Department of
Environmental Protection, State of Maine. 2005. http://www.
maine.gov/dep/dioxin/.

3. id

4 "Xylenes, Hazard Summary." Technology Transfer Network,
Air Toxics Web Site, US EPA.revised January 2000. http://www.
epa.gov/ttn/atw/hlthef/xylenes.html.

5. "Toluene, Hazard Summary." Technology Transfer Network,
Air Toxics Web Site, US EPA. revised January 2000. http://www.
epa.gov/ttn/atw/hlthef/toluene.html.

6. L. Atkinson, P. Ince, N.M. Smith and R. Taylor, Royal
Victoria "Clinical Toxicology: Toxic reaction to inhaled paint
fumes." Infirmary, Newcastle upon Tyne NE1 4LP, UK. http://
www.ncbi.nlm.nih.gov/pmc/articles/PMC2429483/pdf/
postmedj00176-0048.pdf.

7. "Indoor Air Quality in Homes/Residences, Painting and
IAO." US EPA. http://www.epa.gov/iaq/homes/hip-painting.html.

Chapter 8

In Your Environment

Tip 27: Outdoor Air

Outside air is filled with many pollutants and respiratory irritants and can cause problems for many people.

What Can You Do About It?

- ○ Use a personal air purifier. These are the size of a cell phone and are worn on a cord so they dangle below your chin. They help to reduce molds and odors, in particular. Call 1-(800)-787-8780 for information.

- ○ Do your part to clean up the outdoor air by carpooling, riding a bike in clean air areas, and using an electric starter on your barbeque grill instead of lighter fluid and charcoal. Attempt to reduce overall energy needs in your home. Do all you can to help clean up the air in your area and make it better for you and others to breathe.

- If you have pollen allergies: On days with high pollen counts, find things to do inside and don't go out unless it is necessary. Move your room air purifier from room-to-room every six hours so the air in the entire house is cleaner. Go to *www.pollen.com* and enter your zip code to receive a four-day allergen forecast for your area.

Why Is Breathing Clean Outdoor Air So Important?

- Outdoor pollutants can cause chest pain, coughing, shortness of breath, throat irritation, and can aggravate asthma.

- On days when ozone air pollution is highest, stay inside. Ozone has been associated with 10-20% of all respiratory hospital visits and admissions.[1]

- High pollen counts can intensify allergies, asthma, and similar conditions.

- Carbon monoxide, nitrogen oxides, sulfur dioxides, and volatile organic compounds (VOCs) are all outside air pollutants.

- High exposure to carbon monoxide can result in carbon monoxide poisoning, which can cause headache, dizziness, nausea, flu-like symptoms, shortness of breath, chest pain, depression, hallucinations, vision problems, impaired memory and motor skills, and even seizures.[2]

- Long-term exposure to nitrogen oxides can destroy lung tissue, leading to emphysema.[3]

- Sulfur dioxide inhalation can cause breathing problems, sore throats, and permanent lung damage. When it is mixed with water and contacts skin, frostbite may occur.[4] Contact with eyes causes redness and pain. Sulfur dioxide is also the cause of acid rain.[5]

○ VOCs (volatile organic compounds) can damage soil and groundwater and contribute to global warming.[6] Some VOCs or solvents such as benzene, toluene, and xylene are suspected human carcinogens and may cause leukemia.[7]

A Boy Affected by the Smell of Hot Tar on a Roof

Jerry

History:

This seventeen-year-old boy suddenly developed tics and twitches when he was exposed to the smell of hot tar on the roof of his school.

○ He became pale and nauseated and developed headaches.

○ He made strange sounds.

○ Different areas of his body twitched and jerked.

○ Others in the school also became sick from the odor.

○ His classmates made fun of him.

Treatment:

An air purifier in his classroom helped decrease the smell, but Jerry had to leave his school temporarily because the odor could not be eliminated. His symptoms were embarrasing.

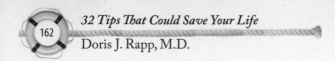
Tip 28: Pest and Weed Control

Pesticides and weed control products used in and/or around the home can cause a vast array of health problems for both humans and animals.

What Can You Do about It?

- Insist on only organic pest and lawn control. Check your local phone book.

- Avoid toxic pesticide sprays used for insect control around the home.

- Learn about safe, effective, and less expensive pest control or IPM.

- Download a free e-book titled *The Bug Stops Here* from *www.thebestcontrol.com*.

- Avoid Organochlorides. This term refers to a wide spectrum of chemicals, including DDT and dioxins. Some organochlorides have been banned in the U.S., but not all. These chemicals are still found in the blood of the vast majority of children and adults.[8]

◦ If pesticide sprays are being applied in your area, do the following:

   ○ Go to another section of town for twenty-four to forty-eight hours.

   ○ Do not allow pets or children outside on the lawn for at least twenty-four hours after the spray.

   ○ If you must stay home, close all doors and windows and turn off your air conditioning. If sensitive, also seal these.

   ○ Use a fan in the bedroom (mosquitoes do not like a breeze).

Why Is It So Important to Use Safe Pest and Weed Control?

◦ Pesticides and other chemicals can be harmful to humans and animals by damaging:

   ◦ normal fetal development;[9]

○ the immune or defense system, leading to more infections, allergies, and cancer;[10]

○ the brain and nervous system, leading to headaches in addition to memory loss, activity, and behavior problems;[11]

○ the endocrine system, leading to diabetes, as well as thyroid and adrenal disease;[12]

○ the reproductive system, leading to increased femininity in males and early puberty in females;[13]

○ the muscular system, leading to muscle aches, fatigue, problems walking, and seizures;[14]

○ the heart and circulatory system, leading to blood clots, irregular heartbeats, high blood pressure, and heart attacks.[15]

These alterations have been linked to multiple sclerosis, Parkinson's disease, and Alzheimer's disease.

- It is possible to become ill from the chemicals (pyrethroids with piperonyl butoxide) used for fogging to kill infected mosquitoes. These chemicals, and those used for killing weeds, can cause asthma, rashes, tremors or spasms, headaches, problems thinking clearly, diabetes, thyroid problems, and cancer. Pregnant rat offspring can have holes in their brains from maternal exposures to chemicals such as piperonyl butoxide. These chemicals also can be toxic to fish, animal wildlife, and birds, as well as humans.[16]

- Chlorinated phenols (organochlorides such as DDT and dioxin) can damage the skin, kidneys, liver, and immune system. Many of these are not only toxic, but are capable of a causing chemical sensitivity illness.[17]

- Leukemia or lymphomas are several times more likely in children if pesticides are used in and around a home.[18]

- Some phenols of the type commonly found in disinfectants can cause genetic

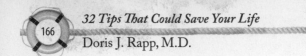
changes and cancer in mammals and are thought to be toxic for the unborn child.[19]

○ Nineteen of thirty commonly used lawn pesticides and twenty-four of forty-eight commonly used school pesticides are probable or possible human carcinogens.[20]

○ Children born to mothers living in pesticide-treated homes during pregnancy have more than twice the normal chance of developing cancer, particularly, acute leukemia or Non-Hodgkin's lymphoma.[21] Some studies show a seven times greater likelihood of developing non-Hodgkin's lymphoma than children who are not exposed to pesticides.[22]

○ When exposed to pesticide use once per week, it is reported that children have four times more chances of developing leukemia and two times more brain cancer by six to seven years of age.[23]

○ Non-organic farmers who use pesticides or herbicides produce more babies with birth defects, have lower sperm counts and testosterone levels, and more depression and suicide.[24]

○ One in 800 non-organic farmers develops cancer. This number drops to one in 20,000 among organic farmers.

Patients Affected By Pesticides

Alice:

○ Fourteen-year-old Alice had extreme reactions to perfume, scented detergents, fabric softeners, paper in new books, mimeographed paper, lighter fluid, lawn chemicals, and asphalt.

○ When she was exposed to these, she babbled incoherently, became giddy, made strange baby talk sounds, and walked and acted in a most unusual manner.

○ These exposures caused her to speak and think unclearly and interfered with her ability to learn and remember. After Provocation/Neutralization allergy treatment she was able to complete college.

○ Once, while walking with her parents, a nearby lawn truck began to spray. Alice became extremely upset and could barely stand up. She had to be supported in order to get home. In another incident, when she walked near a recently pesticide-treated lawn, she suddenly became angry and, again, almost collapsed. She had to be supported and could not walk normally. See www.drrapp.com.

Treatment:

A video clip of Alice's response to one drop of an allergy extract of peas is illustrated on the DVD entitled, *Environmentally Sick Schools*. A number of foods, chemicals, and molds caused similar reactions. With the proper dilution of the offending substance using Provocation/Neutralization testing, her reactions could be reproduced; and with Provocation/Neutralization treatment, her reactions could be prevented or stopped within ten minutes.

Tip 29:
Electromagnetic (EM) Energy

Electromagnetic energy is everywhere and can cause damage to your health.

Who is Most Sensitive to Electromagnetic (EM) Energy?

- Those most at risk are the unborn, the very young, the pregnant, and the elderly.[25]

How and Where Are We Exposed?

- Electromagnetic energy is emitted from cell phones, cordless phones, television cable or cell towers, high-tension power lines, pacemakers, fans, motors, pumps, furnaces, LEDs (light-emitting diodes), and electric blankets.

- We are electrical beings, and our bodies contain water and salt. This means we conduct electromagnetic energy, so we can be affected.

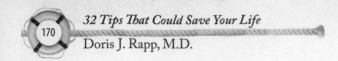

How Can You Tell If EM Energy is Hurting You?

The clue to the role of possible illness related to EM exposure is for you to ask yourself this:

- When was I exposed to more EM than usual and when did I become ill? For example, did you move near high voltage power sources or cables? Were many electric dishes or cable towers erected near your home a few days or weeks before you noted one of more of the symptoms enumerated below?

- Ask if others in your area have recently also developed symptoms. Did their symptoms suddenly begin after the same new EM exposure began to bother you?

What are the Major Symptoms of EMF Exposure?

A very wide array of human symptoms have been attributed to electromagnetic exposure.[26]

Affected individuals will typically have a number of the following complaints:

Headaches, dizziness, memory loss, irritability, depression, anxiety, fatigue, muscle and joint pain, spasms, numbness, paralysis, strokes, insomnia, heart palpitations, irregular heartbeat, increased blood pressure, shortness of breath, sinus problems, asthma, bronchitis, shortness of breath, pain or burning of the eyes, blurred vision, cataracts, skin rash, burning, flushing, itching, miscellaneous testicle or teeth pain, nosebleeds, hair loss, ringing in the ears, thyroid illness.

Numerous Unsubstantiated Medical Claims Attributed to Cell Phones Require More Scientific Documentation

- About 40-50,000 brain tumors and eye cancers per year are attributed to cell phones but many reports disagree with this statement. There is agreement, however, related to the development of acoustic neuromas around the ear after cell phone use.[27]

- Some reports suggest that exposure to banks of computers during pregnancy increases birth defects and miscarriages, but more studies are needed.[28]

- A possible link has been stated between electric and magnetic fields of 60Hz from appliances, house wiring, power lines, and electric blankets and changes in human hormone levels.[29]

- It has been suggested, but not confirmed, that cell phones kept in pants are linked to possible testicular cancer and lower sperm counts.[30]

- One report noted that blood sugar levels rose when EMF exposure or pollution increased. When the offending foods were omitted from the diet, the blood sugar is stated to have stabilized.[31]

What Can be Done To Verify Excessive EM Exposure?

- Measure and compare each room when all electrical things are disconnected, then connected, and again when all electrical appliances. Home kits are available to measure and interpret readings. Call Bau Biologie 727-461-4371. This is an international organization that evaluates EM exposures.

⊙ They can help you with a home evaluation or instruct you in how to evaluate your home on your own. You can acquire meters to measure electromagnetic exposures in every room and outside your home, school, and work areas.

What You Can Do About Illness From Harmful Electromagnetic Exposure?

Even though there are disagreements about safety issues, caution is suggested until we know more.

⊙ Try not to live or work close to high-tension electric wires, TV stations, or cell phone towers.

- If you're exposed to high levels, disconnect or neutralize as many EM energy sources as possible.

- Plug-in filters at outlets reduce exposures (some need ten to twenty per home).

- You can put a button on your cell phone that is claimed to reduce exposure to EM energy. These are obtainable through Naturx at: 480-361-8410 or Bio Pro 1-866-999-2747.

- Try not to use electric blankets or electric heating pads, especially if pregnant.

- The best thing to do if you are seriously ill is to check out some other area that does not cause symptoms. If some area of your city or town is badly polluted with high-tension wires or sources of electromagnetic energy, it is sometimes best to cut your losses and move to a place where you feel fine as soon as possible. Nothing is as important as retaining or regaining your health.

Tip 30: Toxic Dump Sites in Your Town

Living near toxic waste dumps or plants that produce toxic waste can severely damage your health.[32]

What Can You Do about It?

- Check with the Health Department for safe areas to live in your city.
- Try to never live in a moldy home, near an expressway, or over a toxic dumpsite.

Why Is It So Important to Do This?

- Women who live within three kilometers of a toxic dump are more likely to give birth to babies with a deformity or an illness such as spina bifida. The findings were based on a study of mothers and children who lived near twenty-one landfill sites in Europe.[33]

- Children have an increased risk of cancer when living within thirty miles of a nuclear power plant.[34]

- Proximity to plants that irradiate foods or produce dioxin or Teflon™ has adverse effects on children and adults' health.

- The World Health Organization states that 2.4 million people die each year due to air pollution, of which 1.5 million are attributed to indoor air pollution.[35]

Notes

1. Environmental Protection Agency. "Outdoor Air Pollution." 2010. http://www.epa.gov/asthma/outdoorair.html.

2. eMedicineHealth.com. "Carbon Monoxide Poisoning Symptoms." http://www.emedicinehealth.com/carbon_monoxide_poisoning/page3_em.htm (accessed May 8, 2010).

3. Wisconsin Department of Natural Resources. "Oxides of Nitrogen." 2007. http://dnr.wi.gov/air/aq/pollutants/oxides/.htm.

4 Agency for Toxic Substances and Disease Registry. "Sulfur Dioxide." 2007. http://www.atsdr.cdc.gov/mhmi/mmg116.pdf (accessed May 8, 2010).

5. Wisconsin Department of Health Services. "Sulfur Dioxide." http://dhs.wisconsin.gov/eh/chemFS/pdf/SulfurDioxide.pdf (accessed May 8, 2010).

6. Kansas Department of Health and Environment. "Kansas Vapor Intrusion Guidance." 2007. http://www.kdheks.gov/ber/download/Ks_VI_Guidance.pdf.

7. AEA Energy and Environment. *Climate Change Consequences of VOC Emissions*. 2007. http://www.airquality.co.uk/reports/cat07/0710011214_ED48749_VOC_Incineration_-_CC_Report_v3.pdf.

8. Mes, Jos. "Polychlorobiphenyl in Children's Blood." *Environmental Research* 44 (1987): 213-220, http://www.sciencedirect.com/science?_ob=Article URL&_udi=B6WDS-4G3K8RY-6&_user=10&_coverDate=12%2F31%2F1987&_rdoc=1&_fmt=high&_orig=search&_sort=d&_docanchor=&view=c&_searchStrId=1330358960&_rerunOrigin=google&_acct=C000050221&_version=1&_urlVersion=0&_userid=10&md5=eb8b44cead09707ee8bf288491e39513.

9. Colborn, Theo and Coralie Clement. "Chemically-Induced Alterations in Sexual and Functional Development: The Wildlife/Human Connection." in *Advances in Modern Environment Toxicology*, edited by Mehlman, MA, 358-359. (Princeton, NJ: Princeton Scientific Publication, 1992).

10. Vine, MA, L. Stein, K. Weigle, J. Schroeder, D. Dengan, C. K. Tse, C. Hanchette and L. Backer. "Effects on the Immune Systems Associated with Living Near a Pesticide Dump Site." *Environmental Health Perspectives* 108 (2000): 1113-1124.

11. Jacobson, J., et at., "Prenatal Exposure to an Environmental Toxin: A Test of Multiple Effects Model." *Developmental Psychology* 20 (1984):523-32.

12. Porterfield, SP. *Thyroidal Dysfunction and Environmental Chemicals-Potential Impact on Brain Development*. Medical College of Georgia. Agusta, GA. sporterf@mail.mcg.edu.

13. Johnson, Christine. "Endocrine Disrupting Chemicals and Transsexualism." www.transadvocate.org/news/htm.

14. Sherman, Janette M. *Chemical Exposure and Disease Diagnostic and Investigative Techniques*. Princeton: Princeton Scientific Publishing Co., 1994. www.janetsherman.com.

15. Rea, William J. *Chemical Sensitivity*. Vols. 1-4, 1992-1997. CRC Press, Boca Raton, FL.

16. Agency for Toxic Substances and Disease Registry. "Toxicological Profile for Pyrethrins and Pyrethroids." 2003. http://www.atsdr.cdc.gov/toxprofiles/tp155.pdf.

17. World Wildlife.Federation "Detox Campaign Factsheet. Organochlorine Pesticides." http://assets.panda.org/downloads/fact_sheet___oc_pesticides_food_1.pdf.

18. United Nations Environment Programme. "Childhood Pesticide Poisoning." 2004 http://www.chem.unep.ch/Publications/pdf/pestpoisoning.pdf.

19. New Jersey Department of Health and Senior Services. "Hazardous Substance Fact Sheet: Phenol." 2010. http://nj.gov/

health/eoh/rtkweb/documents/fs/1487.pdf; United Kingdom Environment Agency. "Phenol." 2010. http://www.environment-agency.gov.uk/business/topics/pollution/208.aspx.

20. Beyond Pesticides. "Health Effects of Commonly Used Lawn Pesticides." 2005. http://www.beyondpesticides.org/lawn/factsheets/30health.pdf (accessed May 10, 2010); Beyond Pesticides. "Health Effects of Commonly Used Toxic Pesticides in Schools." http://www.beyondpesticides.org/lawn/factsheets/30health.pdf (accessed May 10, 2010).

21. Sinclair Wayne and Richard Pressinger. "Chemical Pesticides: Health Effects Research." http://www.chem-tox.com/pesticides/#birthdefects (accessed May 10, 2010); Beyondpesticides.org. "A Beyond Pesticides Fact Sheet: Children and Lawn Chemicals Don't Mix." 25 (2005): 15-17, http://www.beyondpesticides.org/infoservices/pesticidesandyou/Summer%2005/children%20lawns.pdf (accessed May 10, 2010).

22. Sinclair Wayne and Richard Pressinger. "Chemical Pesticides: Health Effects Research." http://www.chem-tox.com/pesticides/#birthdefects (accessed May 10, 2010).

23. id

24. Agricultural Resources Center and Pesticide Education Project. "Examining the Evidence on Pesticide Exposure & Birth Defects in Farm Workers: An Annotated Bibliography, with Resources for Lay Readers." (2006): 1-21; Perron T, Hernandez AF, Villanueva E. "Increased Risk of Suicide with Exposure to Pesticides in an Intensive Agricultural Area. A 12-year Retrospective Study." *Forensic Science International* 79 (1996): 53-63.

25. International Commission on Non-Ionizing Radiation Protection. ICINRP Guidelines. "Guidelines for Limiting Exposure to Time-Varying Electric, Magnetic and Electromagnetic Fields (Up to 300 GHz)." *Health Physics* 74 (1998): 494-522, http://www.icnirp.de/documents/emfgdl.pdf.

26. Department of Communications, Marine and Natural Resources, Ireland. "Health Effects of Electromagnetic Fields." http://www.dcenr.gov.ie/NR/rdonlyres/9E29937F-1A27-4A16-A8C3-F403A623300C/0/ElectromagneticReport.pdf (accessed May 11, 2010).

27. Christensen HC, Schuz J, Kosteljanetz M, Poulsen HS, Thomsen J, Johansen C. "Cellular Telephone Use and the Risk of Acoustic Neuroma." *American Journal of Epidemiology* 159 (2004): 277-283, http://aje.oxfordjournals.org/cgi/reprint/159/3/277.

28. Kruppa K, Holmberg PC, Rantala K, Nurminen T, Saxen L. "Birth Defects and Exposure to Video Display Terminals During Pregnancy: A Finnish Case-Referent Study." *Scandinavian Journal of Work, Environment & Health* 11 (1985): 353-356, www.sjweh.fi/download.php?abstract_id=2213&file_nro=1.

29. Maisch, Don. "EMFs from Electrical Wiring and Appliances." 2004. http://www.emfacts.com/papers/home_infosheet.pdf (accessed May 45 2010).

30. Morgan LL, Barris E, Newton J, O'Connor E, Philips A, Philips G, Rees C, Stein B. "Cell Phones and Brain Tumors: 15 Reasons for Concern." (2009): 1-38, http://www.radiationresearch.org/pdfs/reasons_us.pdf.

31. Havas M. "Dirty Electricity Elevates Blood Sugar Among Electrically Sensitive Diabetics and May Explain Brittle Diabetes." *Electromagnetic Biology and Medicine* 27 (2008): 135-46, http://www.ncbi.nlm.nih.gov/pmc/articles/PMC2557071/pdf/lebm27-135.pdf.

32. Vine, MA, L. Stein, K. Weigle, J. Schroeder, D. Dengan, C. K. Tse, C. Hanchette and L. Backer. "Effects on the Immune Systems Associated with Living Near a Pesticiede Dump Site." *Environmental Health Perspectives* 108 (2000): 1113-1124.

33. Dolk, H. et al. "Risk of congenital anomalies near hazardous-waste landfill sites in Europe: the EUROHAZCON study." *Lancet* 352 (1998): 423-427.

34. Magnano JJ, J. Sherman, C. Chang, A. Dave, E. Feinberg, and M. Frimer. "Elevated Childhood Cancer Incidence Proximate to U.S. Nuclear Power Plants." *Archives of Environmental Health* 58 (2003): 74-82.

35. Palmer, Sharon. "Irradiation: What It Is, What It Does, and How It Affects the Food Supply." *Today's Dietician* 11 (2009): 32, http://www.todaysdietitian.com/newarchives/011209p32.shtml; Akhmedkhanov A, B. Revich, J. J. Adibi, V. Zeilert, S. A. Masten, D. G. Petterson, Jr., L. L. Needham, and P. Toniolo. "Characterization of Dioxin Exposure in Residents of Chapaevsk, Russia." *Journal of Exposure Analysis and Environmental Epidemiology* 12 (2002): 409-417; Fitzsimmons C. "Teflon Coating Process." eHow. http://www.ehow.com/how-does_5171671_teflon-coating-process.html (accessed May 10, 2010).

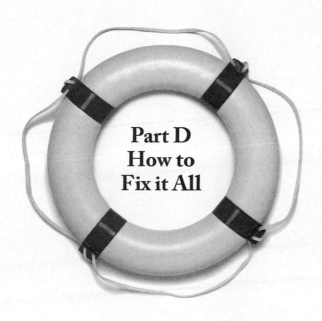

**Part D
How to
Fix it All**

Chapter 9

Cleansing Inside Out

Tip 31: Detoxifying Your Body

The toxins in the environment, in the products you use on or near your body, and in the food you eat can build up in your body over time. We must do all we can to keep toxins and pollutants from entering our bodies, and we must diligently try to eliminate those toxins that have already entered our bodies. This process, is called detoxification, or detox. Harmful toxins enter the body through our food, water, and air. After the toxins leave the intestine, the body's first defense is the liver. In that organ, they either need to be changed so they are no longer harmful or shunted out of the body so the other organs are not damaged. This means that your liver needs a wide range

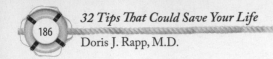
of nutrients so it can properly neutralize and handle the load of pollutants that face most of us on a daily basis. One line of products that contain the types of nutrients your body needs to accomplish better detoxification is available through *www.BodyHealth.com* or 1-877-TO-HEALTH.

We should all eliminate as many of the stored chemicals in our bodies as possible by using the following methods of detoxification.

Check with your doctor if you have kidney, heart, or other serious medical problems prior to beginning any detoxification regimen.

Role of Water in Detox

Drink, drink, and drink—plain water, preferably only from glass containers. This would be well-tolerated and beneficial for many, and it alone appears to relieve some types of chronic illness (arthritis, for example).

How much water do you need to flush out the wastes? One estimate states you should drink half your body weight in ounces each day. For example, if you weigh one hundred twenty-eight pounds, you need about sixty-four ounces, or at least eight full 8-ounce glasses of water every day. If your body is well hydrated, your urine will be colorless or very pale yellow.

Role of Improved Lymphatic Drainage in Detox

Many patients will need to be advised about how to improve their lymphatic drainage since movement or circulation of lymph fluid is an essential adjunct for detoxification or elimination of stored chemicals in the body.

This should also help to prevent and control some infections and can help those with chronic ear, sinus, or lung infections, intestinal problems, or headaches.

There are some simple things you can do to open or drain the lymphatic system in specific problem areas of the body. Many videos demonstrating how to do sinus drainage are

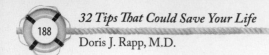

available online, and observing one might be most beneficial for some who have chronic sinus complaints.

One inexpensive way to stimulate the movement of lymph, all on your own, is to walk in such a way that you rock up on your toes with each step. Do this for ten to twenty minutes each day.

○ Massage and Lymphatic Drainage

Some massage specialists also believe that regular lymphatic drainage of the breast and prostate areas will help to diminish the tendency to cancer in these areas. We need research to determine how much this might help.

○ Tight brassieres should be discouraged because they can block proper lymphatic drainage in the breast area and possibly make females more prone to cancer.

○ There are also some relatively expensive machines (such as a chi machine) that, in essence, shake up your lymphatic system so lymph movement and drainage is promoted. They vibrate the entire body, moving the lymph and reducing stress. They also stabilize the skeletal and autonomic nervous system. This improves function of the muscles, stomach, and intestines. Types available include the Evergain and Stressbuster Aerobic Exerciser.

○ Another method uses an expensive electrical device over specific lymph centers to restore and improve lymph flow. In addition, it is said to provide super oxygenation to enhance the healing potential of targeted areas. This is called the ST8 or the Scalar Transmitter Tissue Detoxification System.

○ Women, note that these machines claim to reduce cellulite, which some believe is due to faulty lymph drainage.

○ Lymphatic drainage specialists are in the phone book's yellow pages under "massage," or you can check with a nearby environmental medical physician for a referral.

○ Another do-it-yourself method is to direct the shower spray up your arms and upper body toward your upper right chest. You can also direct the spray up your legs and down your abdomen to your groin area or to the upper right chest. This is the way the lymph normally travels.

Role of Homeopathy or Herbal Remedies in Detox

Single homeopathic items or mixtures of oral herbal or homeopathic detoxification preparations are believed to be helpful and are inexpensive forms for treatment to help eliminate toxins from your body. One relatively inexpensive product by Heel called "The Detox-Kit" appears to be helpful.

Some environmental medical specialists routinely suggest herbal or either single or mixed homeopathic preparations to treat chemical sensitivities. Some of the companies who sell these remedies have studies to help document the effectiveness of their preparations. You can check for their claims and research on their Web sites.

Some homeopathic remedies can easily, effectively, and inexpensively help certain illnesses, especially chronic ear and flu infections and sprains or joint injuries. If these remedies, however, do not quickly relieve an infection, antibiotics should be prescribed. Again, use common sense and check with your physician. In time, more unbiased research will help us to better evaluate what helps and what does not appear to be effective.

In general, homeopathic remedies may or may not help, but they rarely harm unless their use delays the use of emergency treatment, for example, of appendicitis.

Role of Muscles in Detox

The body requires regular and consistent exercise to help muscles contract, which helps

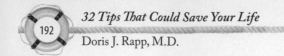

to eliminate waste. The minimum suggested walk time for a normal person without health problems is twenty minutes every other day. If your leg muscles tend to cramp with exercise, have your physician check your red blood cell magnesium levels.

Role of Lungs in Detox

Deeper breathing, with or without exercise, is one simple and excellent way to help eliminate some gaseous or volatile unwanted body wastes via the lungs.

Role of Saunas in Detox

Infrared or other saunas claim to help detoxify or eliminate chemicals and heavy metals, but these are quite expensive. A two-person unit costs about $3000 to $4000. Portable units, however, can be purchased for around $400 to $800. Try to use one that supplies oxygen to the nose and brain because the head is outside the chamber to enhance brain function.

Four cautions regarding saunas:

1. You should be careful of the less expensive plastic sauna versions. They can emit harmful phthalate chemicals when they heat up. These can cause illness for some who are very chemically sensitive. Simply notice if you feel alright after you are in a hot sauna

2. If you have major chemical sensitivities, detoxify very slowly in a sauna or you can become sicker. Do not attempt to do it yourself without experienced environmental medical supervision.
   Call AAEM: 316-684-5500.

3. This form of therapy is sometimes used in conjunction with machines that produce compressed oxygen at six liters per minute. This will enable you to increase the oxygen level in your body cells, including the brain. If your head is inside an enclosed sauna and you are breathing oxygen, you can re-inhale the chemicals that your body excretes. It might be best to use these forms of therapy at different

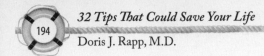

times or use a sauna that allows your head to remain outside.

4. Be most careful of electrical sparks and oxygen! **Check with your doctor before using saunas or oxygen.**

Role of Oxygen in Detox

Increasing the oxygen in your body helps to release toxins from the blood. The simplest form of increasing your body's oxygen is to do deep breathing exercises. Hydrogen peroxide therapy was also a popular form of oxygen detoxing, and many doctors and patients claim it is helpful. However, more scientific documentation is needed.

Role of Liver in Detox

As mentioned before, the liver processes just about everything that enters the body. It is responsible for filtering toxins into the kidneys so they can be expelled from the body rather than being stored in fat. When the body is over-exposed to toxins and chemicals, the liver has a hard time processing all of them, resulting in buildup of toxic substances. Natural liver cleansers include milk thistle, dandelion root, artichoke, and turmeric. These are believed to help the liver to regenerate cells and repair itself. Dandelion root is a natural diuretic and helps clear toxins through urination and also helps stimulate liver bile flow so waste can also be eliminated.

Role of Baths in Detox

Baths are not only great for relaxation, they can be an excellent element in your detoxification regimen. Detox baths help your body to release the toxins built up inside as well absorb the nutrients and minerals in the water.
One cup of either epsom salts, baking soda, or apple cide vinegar or some essential oils can be added to a bath to promote detox. Ginger tea or in the bath water works by heating up the body and causing it to sweat out the toxins. Be careful with the amount added, however, as

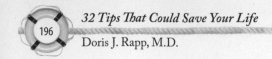

it may turn the skin red temporarily. Always drink plenty of water and have some handy when taking a detox bath.

Role of Bowel Cleansing in Detox

Having regular bowel movements, especially during a detox program, is essential for expelling toxins from the body. An unhealthy colon can cause constipation, gas, bloating, irritable bowel syndrome, headaches, bad breath, allergy symptoms, premenstrual syndrome, fatigue, depression, irritability, frequent infections, and weight gain. Using a colon cleansing kit can be very helpful in a detoxification program. Dr. Natura's Colonix and Toxinout programs are frequently recommended kits on the market, costing about $88.00 for each kit. The products do come with a 60-day money-back guarantee. There are also many colon-cleansing diets that can help. **Check with your doctor for personally designed recommendations.**

For in-depth details and suggestions about different detoxification programs, read Jacqueline Krohn's book, *Natural Detoxification Detoxification* (it is out of print so try Amazon used books).

Role of Nutrition in Detox

While there are a great many methods of detoxifying the body, any regimen will be most beneficial if used with a diet high in fiber, fruits, and vegetables and low in sugar and fat.

Why Is Detoxification So Important?

- The body stores harmful toxins and chemicals. Detoxification helps remove these and also makes one feel healthier and rejuvenated, both physically and mentally.

- Studies show that many of the toxins that build up in the body have been associated with hormone disruption, immune system suppression, reproductive disorders, several types of cancer, and other disorders such as allergies.[1]

✪ One study showed that PCBs (Poly chlorinated biphenols) and DDE (a breakdown product of DDT) levels appear to be unexpectedly high in the general population and may actually be increasing. Regular detox will help to cut down on the level of these harmful chemicals in the body.[2]

✪ Animal and human studies suggest that PCBs can have adverse effects on human behavior,[3] learning, and development, as well as possibly contributing to other types of illnesses, including cancer.[4]

✪ In the bald eagles, the higher the levels of DDE and PCBs in their bodies, the less capable they are of breeding successfully.[5]

Tip 32: Become Pro-active

Becoming pro-active and working to save our planet is something that many people need to do. We need to join together to help the world continue to be a habitable place for generations to come.

The first step to becoming pro-active is to stop making excuses, as legitimate as they may be or seem, for why it is too difficult, too expensive, or simply inconvenient to make changes to your lifestyle so you and your family are safer. There is something that everyone can do at little or no cost.

What Can You Do About It?

- Share information with as many people as possible. Share the problems that concern everyone and suggest what we can do about them.

- We must unite and insist on much less pollution.

Doris J. Rapp, M.D.

- Join "green" and pro-earth organizations to help spread the word. After you join, recruit two friends. Ask them to recruit two friends, and so on and so on. Even this small effort of calling just two people can make a world of difference.

- Drive an alternative fuel, hybrid, or at least highly fuel-efficient vehicle.

- Replace your household cleaners with "green" versions. These are becoming more widely available and are often the same price or even less than the regular products.

- Change the light bulbs in your home to energy efficient bulbs.

- Use solar power as much as possible.

- Ride a bicycle.

- Recycle.

- Plant a tree.

- Educate your neighbors about safe lawn control and the dangers of pesticide use inside and outside the home.

Why is it So Important to Do This?

- We desperately need to protect the next generation. This cannot be done if the present generation continues to ignore the harmful effects of allowing toxins in our food, air, and water.

- We need to protect ourselves and diminish the present day epidemics of illnesses such as cancer, birth defects, ADHD, autism, diabetes, and impotence.

- We need to protect our planet, our wildlife, soil, land, air, and water.

- We must protect the balance of nature because our world has not had the time to adapt and compensate for our gross environmental neglect, irresponsibility, and greed.

Notes

1. Sherry Rier and Warren G. Foster. "Environmental Dioxins and Endometriosis." *Toxicological Sciences* 70)2002): 161-170, http://toxsci.oxfordjournals.org/cgi/content/full/70/2/161#FN1.

2. Ayurdeva, M. "Banned PCBs and Agrochemicals in Blood Reduced by 50%." October 2007. http://www.panchakarma. com/banned-pcbs-and-agrochemicals-in-blood-reduced-50-percent-a-316.html (accessed on June 29, 2010).

3. Vreugdenhil, Hestien J I, Froukje M E Slijper, Paul G H Mulder, and Nynke Weisglas-Kuperus "Effects of perinatal exposure to PCBs and dioxins on play behavior in Dutch children at school age." http://www.ncbi.nlm.nih.gov/pmc/articles/ PMC1241045/.

4. Warner, Marcella, Brenda Eskenazi, Paolo Mocarelli, Pier Mario Gerthoux, Steven Samuels, Larry Needham, Donald Patterson, and Paolo Brambilla "Serum dioxin concentrations and breast cancer risk in the Seveso Women's Health Study." *Environmental Health Perspectives* 110, no. 7 (2002): 625–628.

5. Kozie, Karin D. and Raymond K. Anderson "Productivity, diet, and environmental contaminants in bald eagles nesting near the Wisconsin shoreline of Lake Superior." *Archives of Environmental Contamination and Toxicology* 20, no. 1 (January 1991).

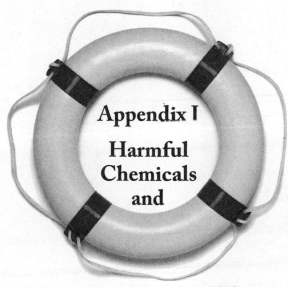

Appendix I

Harmful Chemicals and

Where You May Find Them

TABLE 1
SOURCES OF FORMALDEHYDE

Formaldehyde is a cancer-causing agent found in some unexpected places. You may be surprised to learn that this very harmful substance can be found in

- Adhesives
- Industrial air pollution
- Antifreeze
- Beverages, beer, wine
- Carpets, carpet pads
- Clothing—polyester, synthetic silk
- Construction adhesives
- Dry-cleaning compounds
- Embalming fluid
- Explosives
- Exterior plywood
- Fabric dyes
- Fertilizers
- Furniture cabinets
- Gas appliances
- Gelatin capsules
- Household waxes, oils, inks
- Laminating materials
- Leather tanning agents
- Maple syrup (some varieties)
- Newsprint
- Perfume
- Pharmaceuticals
- Phenol formaldehyde resin
- Photographic chemicals and film
- Plastics, plastic cleaners
- Shoe polish
- Tissues (facial, toilet paper)
- Tobacco, tobacco smoke

TABLE 1

CONTINUED

- Upholstery foam
- Vitamin E and A preparations
- Wallpaper
- Cleaning solutions, detergents, laundry starches
- Cosmetics, mouthwash, toothpaste, deodorants, nail polish, nail hardeners, shampoos
- Disinfectants, bactericides, fungicides, germicides, room and air deodorizers
- Fabrics: wrinkle-proof, water resistant, dye-fast, flame resistant, moth-resistant, shrink-proof, elastic
- Hair growing products, hair setting lotions
- Insect repellents, pesticides, rodent poison

- Jute or hemp fiber preservative (carpet backing, burlap, area rugs, rope, twine)
- Paints, finger paints, enamels, tempera paints, lacquers, varnish removers, wood preservatives, wood stains, wood veneers, particle board, chipboard, interior plywood, wood paneling
- Plaster, stucco, wallboard, concrete, Bakelite, cellophane
- Upholstery fabrics and finishes (permament press, water resistant, dye-fast, flame resistant, moth resistant, shrink-proof, mildew-proof)
- Urea formaldehyde foam insulation (UFFI), glass fiber insulation
- Mattresses (treated with flame retardant)

TABLE 2
SOURCES OF GLYCERINE

Glycerine is sometimes called glycerol, glycol, glyceryl or P.E.G. and can be found in the following:

- Adhesives
- Aftershave lotions
- Antifreeze
- Astringents
- Cosmetics (especially cakes or compacts)
- Cough drops
- Disinfectants
- Dry cleaning agents
- Eye drops
- Fabric softeners
- Face masks
- Fire retardant for textiles
- Flavorings
- Floor polishes
- Food additives
- Freckle lotion
- Furniture polish
- Inks (ballpoint pen, copier, felt tip pen, permanent marker, printer, rubber stamp, water soluble)
- Latex paints
- Leather
- Liquid soaps
- Margarine
- Modeling clay
- Mouthwashes
- Nail polish
- Oven cleaner
- Paper
- Perfume
- Pharmaceuticals
- Plastics

TABLE 2

CONTINUED

- Polishes
- Polyurethane foam (auto dashboards, carpets, flooring, seat cushions)
- Regenerated cellulose
- Saddle soaps
- Shaving creams and lotions
- Shoe polish
- Shortening
- Solvents
- Styptic pencils
- Suntan preparations
- Textile finishes

TABLE 3
SOURCES OF PHENOLS

The following are common sources of phenols, also called phenolics. On food or drink labels, they may be called "flavanoids." The term "phenols" refers to a large spectrum of chemicals including some fungicides, plasticizers (used for hardening or adding shine or pliability to plastics), disinfectants, and antiseptics.

- Acne medications
- Adhesives, glue
- Aspirin
- Bakelite
- Baking powders
- Cannabis (marijuana)
- Caulking agents
- Coal tar
- Creosote
- Detergents
- Disinfectants (pine, such as Pine Sol™ and Lysol™)
- Dyes
- Epoxy and phenolic resins
- Explosives
- Fiberglass
- Flame retardant finishes
- Food additives
- Insulation: thermal and acoustical
- Laundry starches
- Matches
- Metal polishes
- Mildew, mildew proofing
- Mouthwashes
- Nylon
- Paints: enamel, tempera, watercolor
- Perfume
- Pesticides and herbicides

TABLE 3

CONTINUED

- Pharmaceuticals
- Photographic chemicals
- Plastics
- Plywood
- Polyurethane
- Shaving cream and lotions
- Shoe polishes
- Spandex: girdles, support hose, etc.
- Synthetic detergents
- Synthetic fabrics
- TB (tuberculosis) skin test solution
- Tin cans (inner lining)
- Tobacco smoke
- Wood preservatives, sealants, solvents
- Inks: fountain pens, printers, stamp pads
- Phenolic plastics, such as hard saucepan handles

- Molded plastic articles such as telephones and toys
- Aerosols used as disinfectants for odor or mold control
- Jute or hemp fiber preservative: carpet backing, area rugs, rope, twine
- Allergy extracts—preservative in traditional allergy extract treatments
- Preservatives in cosmetics: mascara, liquid eye liner, cream rouges, and eye shadow
- Preservatives in medication: nose and throat sprays, bronchial mists, cough syrup, eye drops, antihistamines, cold capsules, decongestants, first aid ointments

TABLE 4
TYPES OF PLASTICS AND
WHERE THEY ARE FOUND

In general, plastic containers should not be used to store hot liquid, frozen liquids or if the surface is scratched.

**Plastic Category
Recycling Code
Where It's Used**

1
PETE—POLYETHYLENE (TEREPHTHALATE)

Polyester, plastic bottles for soft drinks, thermal insulation, "space blankets," tape, frozen dinner trays, can be recycled into fabric for clothing.

2
HDPE—POLYETHYLENE (HIGH DENSITY)

Laundry soap bottles, milk jugs, storage sheds, plastic bags, chemical-resistant piping, fireworks display mortars, natural gas pipes, water supply pipes, coax cable insulators, refillable water bottles.

3
PVC—Polyvinyl Chloride

Pipes/plumbing, vinyl clothing and records, debit/credit cards, vinyl siding.

4
LDPe—Polyethylene
(Low density)

Food storage and laboratory containers, general storage containers, corrosion-resistant work surfaces, parts that require flexibility, soft and pliable machinery parts, soda six-pack rings, coating on paperboard, aluminum laminated for beverages, computer parts

5
PP—Polypropylene

Plastic hinges, plastic items for medical and laboratory use, Rubbermaid™ and Sterilite™ containers, Under Armour clothing (widely used by the U.S. military), insulating cables, waterproof coating on rooftops, ropes, injectable plastic molds, protective document sleeves, diapers, baby wipes, yogurt containers

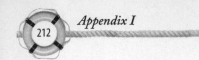

6

PS - POLYSTYRENE

Disposable cutlery, plastic models, CD and DVD cases, Styrofoam™, clear plastic drinking cups, molded parts inside cars, housings for computers, hairdryers, smoke detectors, and kitchen appliances

7

OTHER - (INCLUDES POLYCARBONATE)

Scratch resistant lenses, beverage bottles, baby bottles, electronic casings, bullet proof materials, three- and five-gallon water jugs, nylon, signs, iPod™ cases

WHAT DO THOSE RECYCLING NUMBERS MEAN?

The numbers stamped or imprinted on the bottom of plastic containers in a triangle refer to the type of plastic used to make the product.

#1 and #2 plastics are the most easily recycled and are accepted by most curbside and drop-off recycling agencies.

#3 plastics are recyclable, but may not be accepted by curbside agencies.

#4 plastics are not generally accepted by curbside programs; however, some grocery stores have receptacles for plastic grocery bag recycling.

#5 and #6 plastics are accepted by some curbside recycling programs.

#7 plastic products are not traditionally recycled, though some services are available. Keep in mind that plastics bearing the recycling #7 are categorized as "other" and may or may not contain BPA (Bisphenol-A). Containers made with BPA should never be used to heat food or beverages.

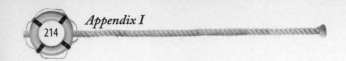

Sources of Bisphenol-A (BPA)

Bisphenol-A, also known as BPA, is a particular phenol used to give strength and shine to hard plastics. It would be virtually impossible to list **all** the consumer and commercial products that contain BPA because the list seems never-ending. In general, hard shiny plastics are likely to contain BPA. Infant care items such as some bottles and pacifiers are among those items containing this toxic additive. Glass baby bottles are best; but opaque hard plastic, non-shiny bottles are reported to be safe.

TABLE 5
INFANT CARE ITEMS THAT CONTAIN BPA

Any infant care product is an especially dangerous place to find a chemical that causes the kinds of damage associated with BPA. The effects of this toxin include breast and prostate cancer, behavioral changes, abnormal development of mammary glands, genital defects and feminization of male infants. BPA-free bottles and pacifiers are essential in maintaining the health of infants.

Many countries have already banned the use of BPA in infant products, and some parts of the U.S. are in the process of doing so, as well.

- Baby bottles and pacifiers (not all—see tables 6 & 7)
- Plastic baby food containers
- Compact disks
- Dentures and other dental devices
- Dental sealants
- Dental composites
- Epoxy resins
- Household electronics
- Impact resistant safety equipment
- Lenses (polycarbonate, scratch-resistant)
- Microwaveable soup packaging
- Plastic dinnerware
- Plastic food storage containers
- Polycarbonate plastics
- Protective linings in food cans (only some manufacturers)
- Refillable beverage containers
- Syringes

TABLE 6
REPORTED BPA- FREE BABY BOTTLES

- Gerber: Clear View and Fashion Tints Nurser
- Evenflo Classic Glass Nurser
- Playtex Drop-Ins
- Dr. Brown's Natural Flow: standard glass bottles and polypropylene plastic bottles (the older plastic model made from polycarbonate is said to contain BPA)
- Green to Grow baby bottles
- Wee Go glass bottles
- ThinkBaby bottles
- Medela bottles
- Born Free: This company makes both BPA-free plastic bottles and traditional glass bottles.

TABLE 7
REPORTED BPA-FREE PACIFIERS

- Natursutten Natural Rubber Pacifiers
- The First Years: Soothies Silicone Pacifiers (including the Soothie Teething Pacifier), Safe Comfort, Ultra Kip, Disney Pacifier, and Attacher
- Vice Versa Binky w/Case
- Playtex: Binky Most Like Mother Latex Pacifier, Binky Most Like Mother Silicone Pacifier, Binky Angled Pacifier, Binky One-piece Pacifier, Ortho-Pro Pacifier
- Evenflo: Mimi Soft Touch, Mimi Premium, Mimi Neo One-Piece, Vizion, Fuzion, and Illuzion
- Gerber: NUK Classic, NUK Original, NUK Nautical
- Happy Baby Silicone Soother
- Nurture Pure Silicone Pacifier
- Born Free Pacifiers

Not every model from the listed brands is free of BPA. Any not listed here must be researched individually to determine whether they contain BPA.

Also note that many of these brands/models claim they became BPA-free in 2008. Be sure that you are using new pacifiers, as those designed and sold before 2008 or early in the year 2008 may contain BPA. Many infant care product manufacturers are planning to be completely BPA-free by 2009, so more choices will be available soon.

TABLE 8
CANCER AND SUSPECT
CHEMICAL CONTRIBUTORS

TYPE OF CANCER	CHEMICAL OR SUBSTANCE
Bladder	Chlorination by-products, cadmium, solvents, diesel exhaust, 4-aminobiphenyl (xenylamine), naphthylamine, benzidine, auramine, magenta
Bone	Fluoride
Brain	Non-ionizing radiation (specifically mobile phones), pesticides, hair dyes, chlordane
Breast	Polychlorinated biphenyls (PCBs)
Cervical	Xenoestrogens (or other feminizing chemicals)
Colon	Chlorine, asbestos (contributes to polyp growth)
Endometriosis	Artificial hormones, Dioxin
Lung	Asbestos (Mesothelioma), cadmium, talc

TABLE 8
CONTINUED

Non-Hodgkin's lymphoma	Benzene (multiple myeloma), lawn sprays and weed killers containing 2,4 D (banned in Sweden, Denmark, Quebec, and Norway).
Ovarian	Talc
Prostate	BPA (Bisphenol-A, found in hard, clear, shiny plastics)
Soft tissue sarcoma	Arsenic, chlorophenols, dioxin, vinyl chloride
Thyroid	High radiation exposure

TABLE 9
EFFECTS OF NAPHTHALENE
(IN SOME MOTHBALLS) ON
HUMANS AFTER CONTACT

Method of Contact Effect on the Human Body

Skin Contact: Skin irritation, severe dermatitis

Acute whole-body reaction in newborns
(less than six weeks old)

Eye Contact: Cataracts, eye irritation

Inhalation/General Contact: Headache, confusion, excitement, nausea, vomiting, sweating, painful urination, blood in the urine, damaged red blood cells.

Complete or partial blindness
(rare but can occur)

Ingestion: Abdominal cramps, vomiting, diarrhea, headache, convulsions, lethargy, sweating, confusion, painful urination, brown or black urine, anemia, fever, jaundice, reduction in kidney function, and liver damage

TABLE 10

THE EFFECTS OF ORGANOCHLORIDES ON THE BODY

FOUND IN	ORGANOCHLORIDE NAME	HEALTH EFFECTS
Solvents	Dichloromethane, chloroform trichloroethane,	Chemical burns may result from skin contact; linked to birth defects and lung, liver and pancreatic cancer as well as heart, lung and kidney abnormalities in lab animals
Pesticides	DDT, dicofol, heptachlor, endosulfan, chlordane, mirex, pentachlorophenol	Exposure is associated with non-Hodgkins lymphoma and liver and pancreatic cancer in humans;
Plastic (PVC/ Polyvinyl chloride)	Vinyl chloride	Angiosarcoma (rare cancer) of the liver, liver damage, production and incineration both form dioxin, which can cause cancer and has been linked to illness in Vietnam War veterans.

TABLE 11

THE EFFECTS OF ORGANOPHOSPHATES ON THE BODY

Trade Name	Organophos- phate Name	Health Effects
Azimil, Bay 9027 & 17147, Carfene, Cotnion-methyl, Gusathion, Gusathion-M, Guthion, Methyl-Guthion	Azinphos methyl	Derived from World War II nerve agents, this pesticide can cause confusion, fatigue, behavioral changes, and degenerative brain diseases.
Brodan, Detmol UA, Dowco 179, Dursban, Empire, Eradex, Lorsban, Paqeant, Piridane, Scout, Stipend	Chlorpyrifos	Has been associated with asthma and reproductive and developmental problems. Babies exposed in the womb have increased risk of developmental delays and behavioral disorders such as ADHD.

Basudin, Dazzel, Gardentox, Kayazol, Knox Out, Nucidol, Spectracide	Diazinon	May cause headache, blurred vision, nausea, chest discomfort, muscle twitching. Severe poisoning can cause convulsions, coma, and death. Causes birth defects and fetal death in lab rats.
Apavap, Cypona, Derriban, Devikol, Duo-Kill, Duravos, Elastrel, Fly-Bate, Fly-Die, Fly-Fighter, Herkol, No-Pest, Prentox, Vapona, Verdisol	Dichlorvos (DDVP)	Can cause central nervous system depression, chest discomfort, unconsciousness, and seizures. Long-term exposure can cause memory defects and delayed reaction times.
Celthion, Cythion, Dielathion, El 4049, Emmaton, Exathios, Fyfanon, Hilthion, Karbofos,	Malathion	Causes skin and eye irritation, cramps, nausea, diarrhea, excessive sweating, seizures, and even death.

TABLE 11
CONTINUED

Bladan M, Cekumethion, Dalf, Devithion, Folidol-M, Fosferno M50, Gearphos, Metacide, Metaphos, Metron, Nitrox 80, Partron M, Penncap-M, and Tekwaisa	Methyl parathion	May cause nausea, vomiting, diarrhea, abdominal cramps, headache, dizziness, eye pain, blurred vision, constriction or dilation of the pupils, confusion, slurred speech, loss of reflexes, weakness, fatigue, paralysis of the extremities, or death from respiratory failure or cardiac arrest.
Rabon, Stirofos, Gardona, Gardcide	Tetrachlorvinphos	Exposure can result in immediate and rapidly escalating symptoms, including headache, sweating, nausea and vomiting, diarrhea, loss of coordination, and even death. Higher exposures can cause accumulation of fluid in the lungs. Repeated exposure may cause personality changes such as depression, anxiety, or irritability.

Table 12
The Effects of Solvents on The Body

Diethyl Ether—Can cause damage to reproduction and birth defects in laboratory animals, headaches, kidney and liver damage. Ether is also highly flammable, even when contacting hot surfaces with no flame, and thus presents a serious fire hazard.

Dichloromethane—Can cause skin irritation, chemical burns. Has been linked to cancer of the lungs, liver, and pancreas in laboratory animals. It crosses the placenta, but effects on unborn are not known. Acetone may cause central nervous system depression and skin irritation.

Chloroform—Immediately dangerous to life and health at approximately 500 ppm (parts per million) according to the United States National Institute for Occupational Safety and Health. Inhalation can cause dizziness, fatigue, and headache. May cause damage to the liver and kidneys. Skin contact can result in sores.

Carbon disulfide—Can cause slight changes in nerves at only 8ppm (parts per million). May cause heart damage in humans. When pregnant rats had breathed 225 ppm, some of their newborns died or had birth defects.

Toluene—May cause cell damage. Low-level exposure can cause temporary tiredness, confusion, weakness, memory loss, nausea, loss of appetite, and hearing and color vision loss. May also affect kidneys. Breathing very high levels during pregnancy can result in birth defects and mental and growth retardation.

TABLE 13
THE EFFECTS OF CARBAMATES ON THE BODY

Trade Names	Carbamate Name	Health Effects
Temik, ENT 27093, OMS 771, UC 21149	Aldicarb	One of the top three most toxic carbamates. Can cause weakness, blurred vision, headache, nausea, tearing, sweating, and tremors in people. May cause death in humans at high doses by paralyzing the respiratory system.
Furadan, Bay 70143, Carbodan, Carbosip, Chinofur, Furacarb, Kenafuran, Pillarfuron, Rampart, Nex, Yaltox	Carbofuran	One of the most toxic carbamate pesticides. One-quarter teaspoon can be fatal in humans. Granular form kills birds after eating one grain.

Fenoxycarb	Comply, Insegar, Logic, Pictyl, Torus, Varikill	Human carcinogen. Suspected of causing birth defects and liver damage.
Carbaryl	Arylam, Bug Master, Carbamec, Carbamine, Crunch, Devicarb, Hexavin, Sevin	Human carcinogen and cause of birth defects and liver damage. Inhalation may cause nausea, vomiting, blurred vision, sweating, and convulsions.

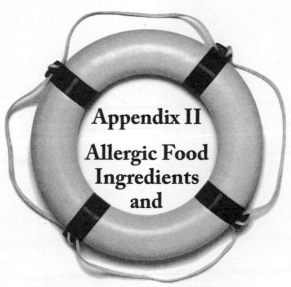

Appendix II

Allergic Food
Ingredients
and

Where You'll Find Them

Allergic Food Ingredients

Many foods such as corn, soy, wheat, eggs, and milk/milk derivatives can cause mild to very severe adverse reactions. In sensitive people, emergency medical reactions can occur even in very small amounts. These tables will help to identify some of the common foods and other items that contain these allergenic substances.

Keep in mind that every type or brand of a listed item may not necessarily contain the allergenic ingredient. Again, always read the labels on food products, especially if you or someone in your household is sensitive to any foods or food additives.

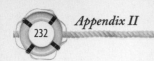

TABLE 14
ALLERGY SYMPTOMS
CAUSED BY COMMON FOOD SUSPECTS

Allergy Symptom	Often Caused By:
Allergic-Tension Fatigue Syndrome	Artificial coloring, cane or beet sugar, milk, corn, cocoa, wheat, corn, oranges, apples, grapes, peanuts, tomatoes, eggs, food additives, artificial flavorings, and preservatives
Aphthous ulcers (canker sores)	Citrus, pickles, apples, coffee, chocolate, cinnamon, nuts, potatoes
Asthma	Milk, eggs, wheat or any other grain, fish or shellfish, peanuts, cocoa, corn, nuts, wheat, onion, garlic
Arthritis	Pork (bacon, ham, etc.), lard, milk, chicken, chocolate, wheat, coffee, eggs, artificial food coloring, corn, fish, turkey, lamb, spinach, cinnamon, and yeast
Colitis	Milk, wheat, eggs, corn, cocoa, nuts, orange, pork, beef, chicken, peanut, sugar
Eczema	Eggs, milk, chocolate, nuts, eggs, peanuts, yeast
Fluid retention	Pork, milk (dairy)

TABLE 14

CONTINUED

Gall bladder disease	Coffee, chocolate, eggs, pork, onion, chicken, oranges, corn, beans, nuts, cheese, and fatty foods
Bladder problems	Milk, eggs, citrus, corn, wheat, pork, tomato, chicken, cola, cocoa, onion, fish, cinnamon, apple, peanuts, fruit juices, artificial color, preservatives
Headache	Milk, chocolate, chicken, coffee, eggs, corn, peanuts, peas, beans, cinnamon, pork, garlic, food coloring, wheat, orange, tea, mushrooms, peas, cane sugar, yeast
Hives	Chocolate, milk (dairy), eggs, peanuts, cinnamon, preservatives, strawberries, melon, tomato, artificial coloring or flavoring or any other food
Otitis (ear infections)	Milk, wheat, eggs, chocolate, peanuts, corn, chicken
Nose allergies	Milk, orange, corn, wheat, artificial food coloring, eggs
Blood vessel disease	Chocolate, corn, nuts, pork, peanuts, coffee, milk, wheat, rice, beef, shrimp or other seafood, chicken, apples (and many chemicals)

TABLE 15
SOURCES OF CORN

- Canned or bottled juice/juice drinks
- Carob (CaraCoa)
- Succotash
- Confectioner's sugar
- Brown sugar
- Corn sugar
- Frostings
- Cornstarch
- Cornmeal
- Candied, canned, or dried fruits
- Frozen fruits (sweetened)
- Fruit desserts
- Cottage cheese
- Ice cream
- Milk in cartons
- Cookies
- Oleomargarine
- Sherbet
- Whole kernel cereal (fresh/canned)
- Yogurt
- Hominy
- Commercial baked goods
- Biscuits
- Cake, pancake and pie mixes
- Donuts
- Corn cereal
- Pre-sweetened cereals
- Candy
- Bacon
- Cooked meats in gravies
- Cured ham
- Luncheon meats (bologna, etc.)
- Sandwich spreads
- Sausages, wieners
- Beer, ale, gin, whiskey
- Corn syrup
- Custards
- Fritos

TABLE 15

CONTINUED

- Graham crackers
- Instant coffee
- Instant tea
- Coffee rich
- Jellies
- Some frozen orange juice
- Creamed pies
- Sorbitol
- Gelatin mixes
- Peanut butter
- Popcorn
- Puddings
- Baking powders
- Corn oils
- Yeast
- Aspirin
- Capsules
- Ointments

- Suppository
- Most tablet medicines
- Bath or body powder
- Paper cups and plates
- Adhesives on envelopes, labels, stickers, tape, etc.
- Liquids in paper cartons
- Some plastic food wrappers
- Toothpastes
- Denture powders
- Gravies
- Monosodium glutamate
- Zest soap

TABLE 16
SOURCES OF SOY

- Soybeans
- Soy sauce
- Worcestershire sauce
- Soy nuts
- Soy noodles, spaghetti, macaroni
- Soy sprouts (Chinese food)
- Tofu
- Infant soy formulas:
- Soyalac or I-Soyalac
- Nursoy
- Isomil
- Prosobee
- Infant milk formulas
- Enfamil
- SMA
- Similac
- Advance
- Portagen
- Alimentum
- Good Start
- Margarine
- Cooking sprays (PAM, Crisco, etc.)
- Crisco shortening
- Ice cream, sherbet, ice milk
- Processed cheeses
- Nondairy products (coffee creamers, etc.)
- Liquid protein foods
- Adhesives
- Blankets
- Candles
- Celluloid
- Cloth
- Cosmetics
- Glycerin
- Linoleum
- Fodder for animals
- Some dog and fish foods

TABLE 16

CONTINUED

- Fertilizer
- Soap
- Automobile parts
- Oils (lubricating)

- Paint, enamel, varnish
- Massage creams
- Paper sizing and finishes

TABLE 17
SOURCES OF WHEAT

- Baked goods
- Biscuits
- Bread crumbs
- Breads (including rye, potato, rice, etc.)
- Breakfast cereals
- Candy
- Coffee substitutes
- Cracker meal
- Crackers
- Dumplings
- Gravy

- Macaroni & other pastas
- Malt (beer)
- Noodles
- Salad dressing
- Sauces for vegetables or meats
- Soups (bisques or chowders)
- Stuffing
- Swiss steak
- Wieners or bologna

TABLE 18
SOURCES OF DAIRY

- Milk (includes powdered, condensed, malted, buttermilk)
- Cream, Half and Half
- Cheese
- Sour cream
- Butter and some margarines
- Whipped cream or topping
- Ice cream/ice milk
- Milk sherbet
- Yogurt
- Casein or caseinate
- Whey or lactose (milk sugar)
- Ovaltine
- Cocoa drinks
- Coffee creamer and substitutes (including nondairy—these can contain casein)
- Some breads and rolls
- Muffins
- Baking powder biscuits
- Pancakes and waffles
- Biscuit or baking mixes
- Pasta and noodles
- Some dry cereals
- Cream of wheat
- Some salad dressings
- Some breaded meats (in coating)
- Creamed meats
- Frankfurters, bologna or luncheon meats containing milk solids
- Creamed vegetables
- Mashed potatoes, potatoes au gratin and scalloped
- Custards
- Cakes
- Puddings

TABLE **18**

CONTINUED

- Cookies
- Cream pies
- Some candies or chocolates

- Bisque or cream soups
- Egg substitutes

TABLE **19**
SOURCES OF EGG

- Albumen
- Baked goods
- Bavarian cream
- Bread crumbs
- Candy
- Coffee
- Creamed foods
- Croquettes
- Crusts (if shiny bread, etc.)
- Custards
- Powdered or dried egg

- French ice cream
- French toast
- Fritters
- Frostings
- Meringue
- Noodles
- Pie filling
- Root beer
- Salad dressing
- Sauces (Hollandaise)
- Sausage
- Soups

More Books by
Doris J. Rapp, M.D.

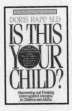

Is This Your Child?

Good reasons it's a NY Times bestseller. It's the only book with a sector on infant and toddler allergies; the hyperactive and aggressive child; the fatigued, withdrawn, depressed, and violent child; Tourette's syndrome; and the the child who simply can't behave.

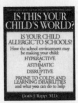

Is This Your Child's World?

This 634-page book holds the keys to not only turn your child's life around, but its practical answers have saved entire families. Your child's world is also your world. Many have tried the suggestions in Chapter 3 and have seen dramatic improvements in just one week.

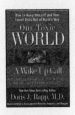

Our Toxic World, A Wake Up Call

Our air, water, food, soil, homes, schools, and workplaces can expose us to chemicals that can potentially harm us. Our Toxic World discusses the abundant evidence of the serious health issues which are becoming increasingly evident as a result of chemicals.

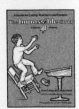

The Impossible Child,
at Home and at School

No, it's not a bad child. Many times it's simply a missed form of allergy that was improperly diagnosed. Learn to spot your child's early changes in appearance, writing, drawing, walking, and speech. How and what can or will the school do to help you?

Visit www.DorisRappMD.com

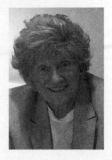

About the Author

Doris J. Rapp, M.D.

Dr. Rapp is board certified in pediatrics and pediatric allergy. She was a Clinical Assistant Professor of Pediatrics at the State University of New York at Buffalo until January 1996 when she moved to Phoenix. She practiced traditional allergy medicine for 18 years; and then, after learning about environmental medicine in 1975, she began to incorporate the principles of environmental medicine in her pediatric allergy practice. She is a certified specialist in Environmental Medicine. She has published 29 medical articles, authored nine chapters in medical texts, and written eleven books and three booklets for the public about allergy. She has also produced numerous educational videotapes, DVDs, and audiotapes for the public, educators, physicians, any others with medical expertise, builders, architects, and lawyers. These demonstrate the dramatic physical and behavioral changes in children and adults that can be produced using this newer, more precise method of allergy testing called Provocation/Neutralization. These newer diagnostic treatment methods can often detect and relieve symptoms in a few minutes. The identical reactions of which patients complain also can be reproduced by asking patients to eat offending foods or to smell offending odors. Single- and double-blinded studies indicate that brain waves, immunological blood changes, psychological tests, writing and drawing, walk and speach can all be dramatically altered during Provocation/Neutralization allergy testing and treatment. It is imperative that both the public and physicians recognize that diverse body areas and a wide range of symptoms can be produced in patients who have unrecognized allergies. The correct diagnosis can be missed for a lifetime because most have no idea that any area of the body can be affected by an allergy or environmental illness. Appropriate P/N allergy treatment for dust, pollen, molds, foods, hormones, and certain chemicals (chlorine, fluoride etc.) appears to be surprisingly helpful in relieving many acute and chronic physical, emotional, and learning problems in both children and adults. See examples at *www.drrapp.com* or on many DVDs taken over a period of 20 years that clearly demonstrate the many ways common dust, mold, pollen, foods, and chemicals can cause illness.

Acknowledgements

This book would not have been possible without the help of my dedicated staff: Jennifer Blevins and Franceska Zweifler, who were masters at creating tables and supplying references and needed patient material, as well as Janyl Tremblay, who provided great assistance for this project.

I am very grateful to each of them for their sincere interest in helping so many families realize the many dangers in and around their homes.

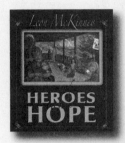
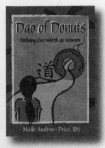
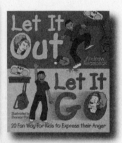
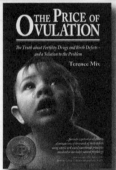
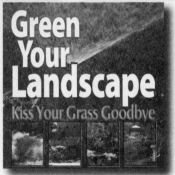